Intercultural Therapy

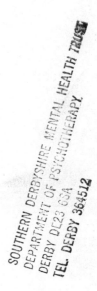

Intercultural Therapy

Themes, Interpretations and Practice

EDITED BY

Jafar Kareem and Roland Littlewood

OXFORD

BLACKWELL SCIENTIFIC PUBLICATIONS

LONDON EDINBURGH BOSTON

MELBOURNE PARIS BERLIN VIENNA

© 1992 by Jafar Kareem & Roland
Littlewood

Blackwell Scientific Publications
Editorial Offices:
Osney Mead, Oxford OX2 0EL
25 John Street, London WC1N 2BL
23 Ainslie Place, Edinburgh EH3 6AJ
3 Cambridge Center, Cambridge,
    Massachusetts 02142, USA
54 University Street, Carlton
    Victoria 3053, Australia

Other Editorial Offices:
Librairie Arnette SA
2, rue Casimir-Delavigne
75006 Paris
France

Blackwell Wissenschafts-Verlag
Meinekestrasse 4
D-1000 Berlin 15
Germany

Blackwell MZV
Feldgasse 13
A-1238 Wien
Austria

First published 1992

Set by DP Photosetting, Aylesbury, Bucks
Printed and bound in Great Britain by
Hartnolls Ltd, Bodmin, Cornwall

DISTRIBUTORS

Marston Book Services Ltd
PO Box 87
Oxford OX2 0DT
(*Orders*: Tel: 0865 791155
         Fax: 0865 791927
         Telex: 837515)

USA
Blackwell Scientific Publications, Inc.
3 Cambridge Center
Cambridge, MA 02142
(*Orders*: Tel: 800 759-6102
         617 225-0401)

Canada
Times Mirror Professional Publishing, Ltd
5240 Finch Avenue East
Scarborough, Ontario M1S 5A2
(*Orders*: Tel: 800 268-4178
         416 298-1588)

Australia
Blackwell Scientific Publications
(Australia) Pty Ltd
54 University Street
Carlton, Victoria 3053
(*Orders*: Tel: 03 347-0300)

British Library
Cataloguing in Publication Data
Intercultural therapy.
  1. Medicine. Therapy
  I. Kareem, Jafar   II. Littlewood, Roland
  615.5

ISBN 0-632-02352-2

Contents

Contributors

Sourangshu Acharyya (MB, MPhil, MRC Psych). Born in Calcutta, India. He trained in medicine and came to the UK in 1974, studied psychiatry at the Bethlem Royal and Maudsley Hospitals and at Guy's Hospital. He has been involved in the development of a community-based Mental Health Centre in South London, and has carried out research into neuropsychiatry, patterns of leadership in multidisciplinary mental health care, on alcoholism and drug addiction. Until recently, he was Research Director at the Nafsiyat Intercultural Therapy Centre. He is an honorary lecturer in psychiatry at University College, London.

Chriso Andreou (BSc, Dip SW, MACP). Worked in Social Services for a number of years before training as a child psychotherapist at the Tavistock Clinic. She is presently working for Wandsworth Health Authority as a Child and Adolescent Psychotherapist and is a psychotherapist at Nafsiyat. She is of Greek–Cypriot origin.

Elaine Arnold (M Phil). Born and educated in Barbados, West Indies. She trained and practised as a Psychiatric Social Worker for several years in Trinidad and Tobago, West Indies and was Co-ordinator of the Community Mental Health Programme. In 1973–75, at Sussex University, Elaine researched into the consequences of the separation and later reuniting of mothers of West Indian origin with their children. Currently she is Tutorial Fellow in Social Work and Social Administration, at Sussex University, and counsellor at Nafsiyat. She has contributed to several training programmes for the statutory and voluntary sectors.

John Bavington (MB, D(Obs)RCOG, MRCPsych) is a Consultant Psychiatrist at Lynfield Mount Hospital where he directs the Transcultural

Psychiatry Unit. He is white, of English/Swiss ancestry. He was born and grew up in the North-West area of British India (now Pakistan). After graduating from London University he returned to work in Pakistan for 17 years, latterly founding and directing the Mental Health Centre at Peshawar.

Jafar Kareem (BSc, MBAP, MLCP). An analytical psychotherapist, a member of the British Association of Psychotherapists and a Training Psychotherapist for the London Centre for Psychotherapy. He has worked in Austria and Israel as well as in the NHS as a psychotherapist, and is an Honorary Senior Lecturer in the Department of Psychiatry, University College. Jafar has been the inspiration behind Nafsiyat and is its founder and Clinical Director. He comes from Calcutta, India, and lives in London. Together with Roland Littlewood he directs the UCL/Nafsiyat Diploma Course in Intercultural Therapy.

Roland Littlewood (MB, D Phil, MRC Psych) is white, of Anglo-Swiss origin. He is a Consultant Psychiatrist, Reader in Psychiatry and Social Anthropology at University College, London, and the author of numerous publications in psychiatry and anthropology including (with Maurice Lipsedge) *Aliens and Alienists*. He is joint-director of the University College Centre for Medical Anthropology, and a past vice-chair at the Transcultural Psychiatry Society. He is currently writing a book, *Pathology and Identity* (Cambridge University Press, published 1992), based on fieldwork in Trinidad with a new religious movement.

Sharon Moorhouse (BSc) is a psychologist and has been carrying out research at Nafsiyat, together with Sourangshu Acharyya, for four years. She is currently writing up an M Phil thesis based on this at UCL and is preparing papers on the work of Nafsiyat. Her particular interest is the development of psychotherapy outside its original social context.

Rosine Jozef Perelberg (PhD) took her doctorate in Social Anthropology at the London School of Economics. She is currently Honorary Lecturer in the Department of Psychiatry, University College, London. Rosine has worked at the Institute of Psychiatry as a psychotherapist and is Senior Psychotherapist and Family Therapist at the Marlborough Family Service. She is a Member of the Institute of Family Therapy, Associate Member of the British Psycho-Analytical Society, and is joint editor of *Gender and Power in Families* (1990). She has directed the UCL Diploma Course in Family Therapy and teaches on the Intercultural Therapy Course.

Derek Steinberg (MB, M Phil, FRCPsych). Consultant Psychiatrist in the

Adolescent Unit of the Maudsley and Bethlem Hospitals in London, and Visiting Reader in Psychiatry and Human Development in the University of Surrey. He is the author of numerous papers and six books on various aspects of clinical psychiatry, staff training, and the organisation and development of treatment services, and he has lectured and taken workshops on these themes in many parts of the world. His grandparents were Jewish immigrants to England from Russia, Poland and Lithuania.

Lennox Thomas (CQSW, MA). An associate member of the British Association of Psychotherapists, a member of The Association for Family Therapy and a member of the Group for the Advancement of Psychotherapy and Psychodynamics in Social Work. He is an external examiner for CQSW Training and is a visiting teacher to the Tavistock Centre. He works as a psychotherapist at Nafsiyat and has been involved in Race and Gender Equality Practice Training since 1981 and is an associate of Freelance Associates for Race Equality (FLARE).

Stuart Turner (ChB, MD, MRC Psych). Studied medicine at Cambridge and is a Senior Lecturer in Psychiatry at University College, London and a Consultant Psychiatrist in North London. He is a medical advisor at the Medical Foundation for the Victims of Torture, and has written widely on the psychological consequences of extreme trauma. He lectures on the UCL Diploma in Intercultural Therapy.

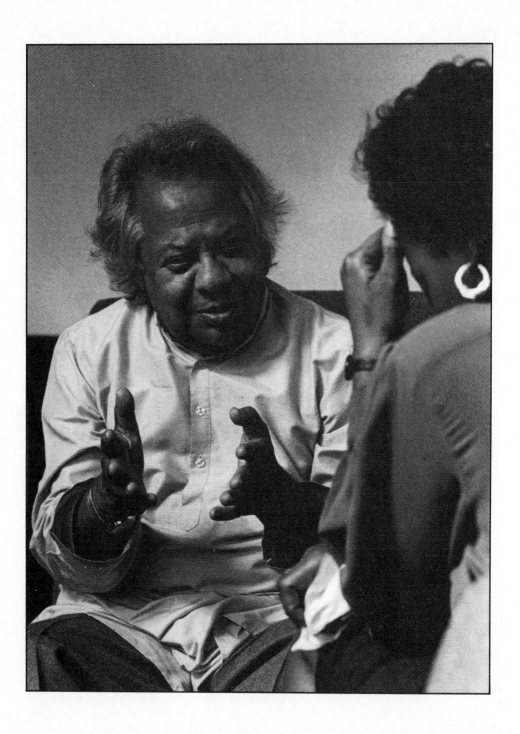

Preface

The idea for this book developed out of discussions at the conference on 'Assessment and Treatment Across Cultures', organised by the Nafsiyat Intercultural Therapy Centre (see Chapter 2) a few years ago. Both editors and all but two of the contributors were involved and continue to work primarily in this field.

The idea for a Centre for Intercultural Therapy came about as a response to the lack of psychotherapy provision for black and other ethnic minority groups. A corollary of this work has been the highlighting of the poverty, deprivation and social powerlessness among many individuals from ethnic minorities and how this can affect their mental health. Much of the work reported here refers also to the inexorable link that is emerging between lack of provision, lack of understanding or misinterpretation (the cases illustrated here will help make this clear) and an increase in social distress.

The book could not have been written, and should not be read, without taking into account the social and political changes that are now taking place throughout Europe. We refer particularly to the re-emergence of extreme forms of nationalism and neo-facism, and the increase in economic inequality and sectarian violence. A recent example in Britain is the Asylum Bill intending to restrict further movement of the migrant population, especially that of political refugees. Although these measures are aimed at curbing abuse of the asylum process, the uncertainty and fear generated does not augur well for the psychological health of Europe. We refer to two effects: fear among the ethnic minority population who have sought refuge far away from their own countries of origin, and guilt, anger and conflict among the dominant group.

Although this volume is grounded in many of the ideas and practices developed at Nafsiyat, we have included pertinent contributions from others involved in intercultural work elsewhere. John Bavington (Chapter 7) works at Bradford, where the Lynfield Mount Hospital was among the first in the UK to consider whether a local minority community could be assisted by a specially focused service. We also include, as a separate Appendix, case examples based on this work; these can be photocopied and used for teaching and group work. Stuart Turner (Chapter 12) contributes his international work with victims of torture and deals here with the topic of the increasing numbers of refugees and migrants to Britain who are the survivors of physical and psychological trauma.

Our book acknowledges the fact that the world – contrary perhaps to the wish of many of its inhabitants, something which is a significant problem in itself – is rapidly becoming a multi-racial and multi-cultural mix. How have we and how do we change to meet that challenge?

A range of different views are represented: we do not believe that there is, or can be, a single model for intercultural work – it is essentially exploratory, essentially a learning process for both sides. In Chapter 1 Roland Littlewood confronts these issues head on, arguing that black and ethnic minority groups have traditionally been denied access to psychotherapy – perhaps for reasons of history since certain specific ideas within psychotherapy derive from nineteenth century Eurocentric ideas. In Chapter 2 Jafar Kareem develops ideas based on experiences within his own analysis and clinical work which have led him to question how universal, and how universally applicable, the procedures of psychotherapy in fact are. Is it really such a 'European therapy' or can it deal with certain basic assumptions about human personality and action? Is it possible to work cross-culturally and if so how? Chapter 3 (Littlewood) summarises recent debates that argue for common characteristics among therapeutic systems and notes how our very definitions of 'problem' and 'treatment' can shift in response to different social and political contexts.

In Part II of the book, with Chapter 4 (Derek Steinberg), we widen the frame still more to examine ourselves in the light of interdisciplinary and interprofessional consultation – indeed the nature of the consultation process as one which includes the client. Steinberg takes us through what is in fact a holistic learning process: what is the patient's own understanding of their difficulties? Chapter 5 (Acharyya) argues that the prevalent model of mental health care confuses the distinction between race and culture looking only at the social creation of distress (and its popular expressions) thus proliferating an ever-widening group of 'medicalised' categories. If the articulation of distress in Europeans (seen through the European-derived model) is seen as universal, indeed 'real', minority and Third World groups then merely have 'local syndromes' – their culture becomes their diagnosis. What a problem we create – the doctor's traditional dilemma – which is the best diagnostic pigeon hole?

In Chapter 6, Sharon Moorhouse summarises her research on the work of Nafsiyat, making the point that no therapist or therapeutic group can expect to be supported unless they can demonstrate that there are tangible gains in terms of psychological and social adjustment for those who come to be healed, and that these gains should be quantifiable against other therapeutic and medical models.

'Practice', Part III, forms the main section of the book. Rosine Perelberg (Chapter 8) takes an anthropological view and discusses the concept of the 'family map' as a formal process of examining how different families live and operate through a world of cultural meanings and constraints.She further suggests that we *can* operationalise such cultural constructs. Chapter 9 (Lennox Thomas) picks up on the work of Chapter 2 to show that any attempt to ignore social organisation and conflict and their representation within our psychology leaves therapy ill-equipped to deal with the problems both of the individual client and of society at large. Thomas points out racism's similarity with sexism – gender difference as power – to argue that to be blind to the meanings of gender or race is to be blind to one's own self – noting the wider implications for therapists in training and for training programmes in general.

Chapter 10 (Chriso Andreou) starts from a more formal psychoanalytical position, describing work with children which integrates external and personal worlds. Her own position as a white therapist with black children, and as a Greek with Turkish children, presents re-enactments of previous social relations and how the images which the dominant society imposes on minority children and their families become a part of their psychological structure. In Chapter 11, Elaine Arnold examines how social workers make assessments of black clients using popular understandings of distress. She goes on to describe the 'forbidden topic' for both black and white – that of children coming to the UK to join mothers whom they have not seen for many years.

In response to the multi-ethnic and multi-cultural community that now is the UK, we have had to learn a lot. Both workers and clients have had to challenge their implicit assumptions about what is internal, private and psychological, and what is external, political and social. Bringing together different perspectives while keeping some overall coherence has been a tough editorial task. We are extremely grateful to all the authors for their ready co-operation; to Richard Miles and Ann Morris of Blackwell Scientific Publications for their patience and advice and to Sally Crawford our editor at Blackwells; to the editors of *Journal of Social Work Practice* and *Holistic Medicine* (now continued as *The Journal of Interprofessional Care*) for permission to include sections from papers which previously appeared in their journals – and which here form part of Chapters 1 and 3 – and to John Bavington for allowing us to develop and use the case exercises from his team.

Sincere thanks also to Yvonne Wright, our secretary at the Nafsiyat Centre, for her patience and cheerfulness throughout the typing and re-typing of the manuscripts. In spite of this arduous and frequently boring task, she has done a marvellous piece of work. We would also like to thank Katy Lawrence, the Administrator of Nafsiyat, and Sharon Moorhouse, its Research Associate, who went beyond their usual responsibilities to provide support and help in the preparation of the manuscripts. Particular thanks go to Heloise Kareem who read and re-read the manuscripts and edited Jafar's paper so many times.

Nafsiyat itself could not have continued its work without the support of a number of bodies, and we owe a particular debt to the Islington Health Authority (now Bloomsbury and Islington Health Authority), Islington Borough Council, the Department of Health, the Mental Health Foundation, and the London Boroughs' Grants Unit. Without our patients this book would never have been written: from them we have received much confidence and encouragement as well as criticism.

Jafar Kareem
Roland Littlewood
London, November, 1991

Part I: Themes

Chapter 1

Towards An Intercultural Therapy

ROLAND LITTLEWOOD

Figures from the UK Office of Population Censuses and Surveys (OPCS) estimate that in 1990 there were over two and a half million people in Britain whose ethnic origins were the New Commonwealth. Together with migrants from the Irish Republic and mainland Europe (and their children), they comprise around 10% of the UK population. While the popular perception among the white UK population is of 'black immigrants', it is as well to bear in mind while reading this volume that perhaps half of all the black people in Britain are British-born. The majority of immigrants to Britain throughout recent history have in fact been white (Littlewood and Lipsedge, 1989).

People from ethnic minorities living in Britain, particularly those who are black, experience a variety of practical disadvantages, particularly in the areas of housing, education, health and employment. They can also be subject, in numberless everyday contexts, to the potential experience of overt racism and prejudice in their face-to-face encounters with the indigenous white population. Although there is little statistical information about their general psychological adjustment, ample evidence has accumulated, especially over the last few years, to show that to be black in Britain today is to be exposed to a variety of adverse stimuli which can add up to a quite serious hazard to mental health. While these may be in part the consequences of selective patterns of migration for the generation who immigrated, and due in part to overtly racist politics where these exist, they can also be related to certain specific patterns of psychiatric intervention (Burke, 1984; Littlewood and Lipsedge, 1989; Lewis *et al.*, 1990) and these will be examined below.

When examining the rates of serious mental illness such as schizophrenia and manic-depressive psychosis (as assessed by hospital admission figures), these appear to be higher on average for immigrants from Northern Ireland, the Irish Republic and the West Indies; hospitalisation figures for British-born

3

African–Caribbeans are even higher than those for their migrant parents (Littlewood and Lipsedge, 1989). The issues, therefore, seem to be not simply those of geographical and cultural dislocation and adjustment or the inevitable stresses of migration. There is also the issue of an ongoing response by the white host society and indeed response *to* the host society and its values and institutions.

There have been various debates in the literature and in the media on the issue of 'misdiagnosis' of mental illness. These are not of primary concern here, except to emphasise that what many professionals, doctors and social workers take as 'unintelligible' and thus 'insane' may, at another level of understanding, be seen as legitimate and coherent human responses to disadvantage and racism. To recognise this is not to see black Britons as helpless pawns, controlled by others, but to recognise that their lives are lived through and against such overarching structures: the experience of being perceived and classified by a set of assumptions and institutions which serve the interests of the dominant group (Littlewood, 1980).

The psychological adjustment of European as opposed to non-European migrants and their children has not been the subject of such medical interest and that in itself is perhaps a matter for concern. Racism based on 'colour' may be less evident here, but we are still working with communities which have also experienced dislocation, adjustment to a new physical and psychological environment and often to a new language and new values. These communities continually have to weigh the success of adaptation against their expectations and there is now a second and third generation growing up who are 'British' and who define their personal goals through those both of their parents and of traditional British society.

How helpful have the mental health and social services been in dealing with intercultural malaise? Professional interest has tended to focus on severe mental illness, rather than on 'psychopathology' in a wider sense – that is, on problems of identity, adjustment, achievement, self-actualisation, personal loss, conflict and resistance. Within the black population, we do know that hospitalised black patients are two to three times more likely to be involuntary patients under the Mental Health Act. In relation to their numbers within the general population, black people are over-represented in psychiatric hospitals, particularly in locked facilities and 'special hospitals', and in probation services and prisons. We also have some evidence that they receive higher dosages of drugs and are more frequently given physical treatments such as electro-convulsive therapy independently of their actual diagnosis (Littlewood, 1986; Littlewood and Cross, 1980).

In contrast to this, there is overwhelming anecdotal evidence that psychotherapy – in either hospitals or outpatient clinics – is seldom offered to black and ethnic minority groups. I use the term 'anecdotal' for I have yet to come across any traditional psychotherapy service which publishes figures on the ethnic background of its clients in relation to the population from which they are drawn, far less providing a statistical account of the efficacy of its work with them. Many British psychotherapists privately suggest that therapy is not appropriate for minority groups because of their supposed lack of 'verbal facility' or the ability to understand and 'work through' their problems in a way that accords with the psychological model.

Why should this be? Let me state at the outset that this volume is not intended to be an experience in self-castigation or catharsis (for authors or readers), but has come about because, as therapists, we recognise that we have long found ourselves dissatisfied with what we offer. To some extent this is a problem beyond the remit of traditional psychotherapy. It is one that is generated in our social structure and in the power of our institutions. It is, nevertheless, let us be honest, in part our own creation and therefore our responsibility. Some of the reasons for this need to be examined a little more fully, for they are likely to be reflected in any future work we do with our own clients, irrespective of our own skin colour, and they will take institutional form in the organisation of psychiatric, medical and social services, and in our public policies.

An international context

To a certain extent the psychotherapeutic neglect of minority groups is a particularly British phenomenon. In the United States, while the black American community has certainly been ignored therapeutically (with a few notable exceptions), much theoretical and practical effort has gone into questions of individual and family therapy for immigrant groups from Europe, Vietnam and Japan. We can now find many practical American texts with titles such as *Family Therapy with Minorities* (Ho, 1987; Gaw, 1982; McGoldrick *et al.*, 1982). This reflects the fact that the United States, unlike Britain, has considered itself explicitly as a country of immigrants, whatever the ideology – pluralistic or 'melting pot', for example – it happens to employ. Outside the USA and Britain, there is the work of Parin and his colleagues (1971) who use traditional psychoanalytical techniques with local communities in Senegal; Wintrob and Harvey (1982) in Liberia; André (1987) in Guadeloupe, and Chiape and Lemlij (1985) and others in Peru. These are not merely sociological and social anthropological studies using psychodynamic interviews, but traditional clinical psychoanalysis. In the United States, the French–American psychiatrist, George Devereux (1970), has carried out psychoanalytical work for many years among the native American community, and there was even a period when anthropologists and social scientists were considered to be ill-trained for their work unless they had undergone a personal analysis (Wallace, 1983). In addition, the studies of Mead, Kluckholn, Benedict, and Erikson (sometimes called 'the Culture and Personality' school), are well known to culturally orientated psychotherapists. The only British equivalent of the use of psychodynamic techniques as a sociological or therapeutic tool with non-Europeans is the work of W.H.R. Rivers (1924), who died in the early 1920s, and whose work is now largely forgotten by most British psychoanalysts (Slobodin, 1978).

A British context: power and prestige?

Let us now turn briefly to the specific questions raised by neglect in Britain of intercultural therapy: first the wider social and political issues, then those issues which seem specific to the practice of therapy itself.

We live in a society in which access to health resources is determined in part by wealth and education, and in part by issues of racial identity as defined by the wider society. The black community in Britain, African–Caribbean and South Asian, is predominantly working class, and is thus faced with the double disadvantage of relative poverty as well as discrimination. Access to time-consuming and costly therapy is less available: just one aspect of a general package of disadvantage that includes poor ante-natal care, scholastic failure and poor housing. If you happen to be black you need to have relatively more wealth to achieve the same quality of life as your white colleagues; black minority groups also remain under-represented in the upper reaches of the health-related professions.

One outstanding exception to the above appears to be medicine. Over a quarter of British doctors qualified in the Indian sub-continent (Littlewood and Lipsedge, 1989). They are particularly well represented in psychiatry and other mental health areas: comprising, according to a study ten years ago, nearly a half of all junior psychiatrists. Arguably, this situation arises because psychiatry is hardly considered to be a particularly 'prestigious' speciality. Why, then, have these working psychiatrists not pushed for psychotherapy for their compatriots? The common response by white doctors to this question is that 'Asians' (I employ the term that is commonly used) are just 'not interested' in psychotherapy; whether as doctors or patients, they are somehow more 'physical', less verbal, preferring, as doctors, to use physical methods of treatment, in other words the sharper end of psychiatric facilities; as patients, on the other hand, they seem to manifest 'hysterical' or 'somatic' symptoms rather than genuine psychological problems (Carstairs, 1973; Leff, 1981).

To take doctors first, it is worth noting that medicine is a notably hierarchical profession in which your immediate superior determines your future career to a considerable extent; becoming even a junior psychiatrist is demanding enough without expecting this particular group of trainee doctors to stick their necks out politically. Doctors trained in South Asia have traditionally been given jobs in the peripheral British hospitals rather than in the more prestigious teaching hospital departments and often specialise in psychogeriatrics and mental handicap. They may have limited access to psychotherapeutic training, to university libraries, or to the sort of intellectual climate in which the value of psychotherapy is taken for granted (Littlewood and Lipsedge, 1981; Anwar and Ali, 1987). Where there are the right opportunities, Asian psychiatrists have taken up psychotherapy as enthusiastically and successfully as their white colleagues: so much so that it is now said that they are spending their time doing psychotherapy as a 'soft option', instead of more serious academic research!

There are few trained African–Caribbean psychiatrists, partly because those doctors who did leave the West Indies tended to go to the United States or Canada. There is also the great difficulty for British blacks in entering medical schools to be considered. Recent investigations at St George's Hospital, for example, have shown that not only academics' decisions but even the computer program were biased against accepting medical students who were black (or, incidentally, who were women) (Commission for Racial Equality, 1988).

I do not intend to detail other professions which practise psychotherapy, except to say that I think broadly similar considerations apply to clinical psychology (Guthrie, 1975). In addition, every black social worker I have worked with has had the experience of being 'expected' to be especially concerned with black clients (clients who themselves are defined, as we shall see, as non-verbal).

Before turning to the process of therapy itself, it might be useful to consider the people who practise it, the psychotherapists themselves. The theoretical centre of psychoanalysis in Britain was effectively the creation of immigrants from Central Europe; many of the classic papers were based on intercultural cases, for example, Freud's 'Wolf-Man' (Gardiner, 1972). Why then did psychotherapists not address the question of therapy across cultural and racial groups in this country? The social and economic history of psychoanalysis in Britain has still to be written, but a start has been made by some analysts themselves (King, 1989; Steiner, 1989). I think that it is significant that many of the psychoanalytical immigrants were of Jewish origin (Gay, 1987), and that they entered a society which (as we have now conveniently forgotton) was rabidly anti-Semitic. In the 1930s the British Medical Association, in an urgent report to the government, opposed the entry of Jewish refugee doctors to Britain (Littlewood and Lipsedge, 1989). A psychotherapy which was able to ignore social contexts in favour of intrapsychic factors alone was clearly safer for the practitioner, and helped establish psychoanalysis as a universal (and thus a 'scientific') process rather than as a culturally 'Jewish' therapy (Littlewood, 1989). At the same time, this particular immigrant group, upper middle class and cosmopolitan, formed links with the intellectual bourgeoisie of North London from whom a considerable number of its patients were drawn. Psychotherapy is, in this context, a private contract between analysand and therapist; the issue of payment was regarded as integral to the therapeutic process and a personal contract between individuals which conveniently allowed any question of the institutional politics of race to be set aside or ignored.

Professional issues: political and therapeutic 'resistance'

We can now address the problems which lie within the therapy and practice of therapy. A common statement, perhaps more muted recently, has been that psychotherapy is essentially culture-bound, if not to the Jewish community, then to the Western bourgeois milieu in which it developed. It is practised by these classes themselves among themselves, and it is thought not to be appropriate for 'non-European' patients, who are regarded as less verbally sophisticated and less 'psychological', who resist dynamic interpretations, and who prefer to express their distress through a different idiom, whether somatic or religious (an example can be found in Carothers, 1972).

These notions can be teased out further. On the question of 'non-European', we are, of course, not talking here of small-scale, 'traditional', peasant, or tribal societies, but of groups within British society, which now form part of our nation. It would be surprising if the children of migrants to Britain, whatever their parental origins, remained unchanged, living as they are, in Western industrialised society, speaking English from infancy, bound to its economic and social structures (with their ever-present representations in advertising, the media, and so on) and able to maintain some type of autonomous prior system of 'traditional' personal identity, self-perception and social relations. 'Culture' cannot be thought of as a bag of memories and survival techniques which individuals carry about with them and of which they have forgotten to divest themselves. Rather it is a dynamic re-creation by each generation, a complex and shifting set of accommodations, identifications, explicit resistances and reworkings. The West Indies, one of these pre-migration cultures, has itself developed as a part of Western society and of the Western political system, one in which aspirations, ideals, goals and notions of personhood are the same as those of the white community in the United States or Britain.

The question of 'non-verbal' has always been a commonly perceived attribute of sub-dominant groups, including women and the working class (Gilman, 1985). The study of popular conceptions of personhood, distress and illness has, however, moved beyond one of a simple binary distinction between Western societies (seen as psychologised and ego-centred) and non-Western societies (seen to have a collective consciousness in which a conflict is expressed through religious rituals or somatic experience such as hysteria and hypochondriasis). We now know from the work of critical psychologists like Rom Harré (1983) or social anthropologists like Arthur Kleinman (1988), that there are many different dimensions of personhood. These include such parameters as public and private; external and internal; objective and subjective, that do not easily fall into typological categories. These can themselves be combined in different ways to give a unique notion of the self for the particular group: they may be manifest as personal psychology (or indeed as physiology), perhaps as moralities and cosmologies (whether these are refracted through shamanism, psychoanalysis, or biomedicine). Some of these 'sociology of knowledge' approaches seem now to be influencing psychotherapy, particularly in the work of Bob Hobson (1986) and David Grove (1989) which use the client's own explanatory models of distress to develop therapy in the individual context.

We also know that our systems of lay psychology – our personal understandings – are neither fixed nor rigid, for they are contingent on context (Littlewood, 1990). We use different aspects of our personhood in different situations (see Chapter 3). This suggests that we have to examine the particular context of the patient/therapist interaction in some detail: what we might not unreasonably term the 'politics' of the therapeutic encounter. While it seems that South Asian-born patients may demonstrate psychosocial distress to their general practitioners in somatic terms more often than do white natives (Bal, 1984), we have to take into account the expression of distress outside the consulting session, to, for example, strangers, colleagues, families and self (Beliappa, 1991). In any situation, certain norms of appropriate self-disclosure, power, expectations of responsibility, and the possibility of action, are, of course, part of 'the patient's conception' of what should happen, and which thus reframe experience and communication. A working class Asian patient is hardly likely to be more than dimly aware of the possibility of formal psychotherapy, and is neither going to request it nor present personal distress in a way that persuades doctor, probation officer or social worker to consider it to be an appropriate option.

What then are the factors internal to therapy itself which often cause white therapists with black clients (or black therapists with white clients) to give up in distress? I think one should not underestimate the historical origins of psychoanalysis, and thus the dynamic psychotherapies in general, and their effect on 19th century developmental theory (Wallace, 1983; Littlewood, 1989). Freud's innovation was to unite in a single idiom both phylogenetic and individual development, generating an evolutionary model which traced our development as persons in parallel with the conjectural psycho-history of humankind in general. Thus there appeared certain formal analogies between the archaic and historical, the non-European, the infantile, and the neurotic. The overtly racist implications of this have now been quietly abandoned, although it is worth recalling Jung's advice to white American therapists in the 1920s that 'the American black has what he calls probably a whole historical layer less' and that 'living with barbaric races exerts a suggestive effect on the laboriously tamed instincts of the white race and tends to pull it down' (cited in Thomas and Sillen, 1972).

If the editors of this book felt that a psychodynamic therapy necessarily implied a position such as the above this book would hardly have been written. Nevertheless, the continuing implications of the developmental model must be borne in mind. What does the particular notion of 'maturity', as used by psychotherapists, actually constitute? The Protestant ethic? Middle-class autonomy? The self-sufficient entrepreneur? Stoicism and deferred gratification? I think it is no coincidence that the sort of therapy which has been most successfully elaborated in work with minority or disadvantaged groups in the United States, such as Salvador Minuchin's family therapy, eschews individual developmental notions in favour of an approach derived from a family's shared values understood through systems theory (Minuchin, 1972).

It now seems likely that it is through family therapy in particular that ideas of selfhood and identity, other than those of the white middle-class, can most successfully be employed by therapists in facilitating change (Littlewood, 1989). By contrast, many individual therapists, by training, inevitably rely on an evaluative rating of psychological defence mechanisms, most of them perceived as inherently maladaptive or at least undesirable. The bodily representation of distress is hardly regarded with approbation. To an extent, then, certain theoretical notions of individuation or autonomy are Euro-centric or at least 'modern'; they can also be termed industrial, bourgeois or 'Western'.

This is a question which has received excessive prominence in the current debate for, to reiterate, we are not concerned in Britain with providing psychotherapy for some hypothetical Third World community; we are talking of ourselves. We are talking about a proportion of citizens in Britain now, a disadvantaged group certainly, but emphatically not one which has some sort of exotic system of psychological and personal development. The notion that Pentecostal churches or Sufi groups *necessarily* provide more effective therapeutic intervention than formal psychotherapy (Calley, 1965;

Kiev, 1964b) is dubious. They may well do so at present, but that is perhaps more to do with the psychotherapist's neglect of the issues, whether this is due to benign indifference or even frank aversion.

The work of intercultural therapy

If we suppose that intercultural therapy – effective therapeutic intervention and facilitation by a member of one ethnic group in the decisions, choices and subjectivities of a client of another – is possible, what are the personal impediments which we may bring, unrecognised, to such encounters? How are the institutional structures of racism reflected in the transferences and counter-transferences of individual clinical practice? When does 'political' resistance become 'therapeutic' resistance?

Consider what happens when a white client sees a black therapist. This is a situation in which we can recognise, even before they start working together, what sociologists call a 'status contradiction'. This may be especially true for the therapist: he or she is a member of a disadvantaged group, from whose position in the social system the white client may already gain economic and status advantages outside the therapy. Yet at the same time the therapist is apparently there to assist, to use their skills to direct a successful interaction with the white client. To heal. As a white person, I often have the experience of being approached by white patients who have previously had a black therapist or doctor, and who now immediately tell me how good it is that I at least am white, as if thereby I have the inherent ability to help them. They are puzzled when I return again to this assumption, one they see as obvious, but which I take (among other things) as an aspect of their current inability to take control of their lives, to work through their personal problems, and in which the past therapy and the black professional is perceived as a transient obstruction, now passed.

The issue of race is rarely absent from therapy even when one shares a client's cultural and ethnic identity. In that sense there is nothing 'special' about intercultural therapy with, say, a black client and a white therapist. In our current situation, I as a white therapist certainly have to consider my own motives in deciding sometimes to work with minority clients, for this is not yet accepted as simply part of what we do. Fifteen years ago my supervisor at the Tavistock Clinic used to tell me that I had chosen black patients precisely because the difficulties of working with them were so great that I would not have to deal with the problem of success, that is, with an independent ex-patient who no longer needed me. And thus, I was told, I could always feel 'needed'. Overstated? Perhaps. Prejudiced? Certainly. And yet I do have to take into account the approval or derision of white colleagues who see me as working with supposedly 'difficult' patients; it is all too easy to develop some patronising assumption of particular skills, of doing a special favour, of relating all therapeutic encounters to some esoteric knowledge of the others' 'culture' (Collomb, 1973).

Every now and then a black patient is referred to me who comes from outside my health authority's local area. There is usually some supercilious comment that I will surely 'find this cultural problem of interest'. Such patients frequently turn out to have quite intractable personal circumstances, severe personality disorders, or to be just rather difficult people. Individuals in other words. The 'difficult' becomes transformed into the 'culture', the personal into the public, the psychological into the political. While it can, of course, be said that a good deal of valuable intercultural therapeutic work of all types is being carried out in a number of settings, it is significant that our failures in practice are ascribed in this way to 'culture', in a fetishisation of difference. This compounds a more general picture in which perception of a minority group as 'having' a problem insidiously turns to perceiving them as 'being' a problem. Thus their culture is held to be good for 'them', bad for 'us'.

When both therapist and client are black the 'status contradiction' still occurs. The client's initial response may be that they are being given inferior treatment or, given the obvious scarcity of black therapists, that they have been 'ethnically matched' or 'specially chosen' in some way. The question of ethnic matching has recently come to prominence in the areas of adoption and fostering, and indeed, more generally, in social work. I certainly think its position needs to be taken more sympathetically by its more liberal critics than previously, but it should be considered as one possible option, rather than 'the solution', one possible choice, analogous perhaps to women's therapy groups. It may present a safe space, but it may also be seen as the convenient excuse for white therapists not to confront their own implicit prejudice, and not to start working with black clients. For 'they' already have their therapists.

Segregation and matching of this type have an attraction in their simplicity. I consider this to be a false simplicity in our situation of muddle and confusion, of coalescences and contradictions, in which we apparently still search for therapeutic encounters, devoid of social constraints, in which 'real work' can be done. Intercultural therapy should never be allowed to become some specialised psychotherapy, to be targeted at black people, but simply therapy which takes into account these issues. Let me add, however, that if I were black I would start by looking for a black therapist; not because of some inherent racial understanding, some shared mystique of consciousness, some hypostasised culture, but because, by and large, black therapists have actually given more serious consideration to the issues.

I would like to end this introductory chapter with a warning. Simply because black people have experienced the sharp end of psychiatric and social work interventions, and because we live in a society in which psychotherapy is perceived as empowering the client, we cannot assume that an adequate or appropriate goal is simply to provide 'therapy'. Psychotherapy is perhaps less innocent and less free of social and political ideologies than is biomedicine; it is potentially far more insidious an agent of social control than is the Mental Health Act itself (Sedgwick 1982; Baron, 1988; Cocks, 1985; Maranhão, 1986). There is, of course, nothing inherently disreputable about 'social control': it is the process by which all societies reproduce themselves through inculcating shared values and behaviour. The question rather is, 'control of whom, by whom and for what end?' We need, not simply 'therapy', but a self-reflexive practice which examines its own prejudices, ideology and will to power, which is aware of the ironies and contradictions in its own formation, and which is prepared to struggle with them.

Chapter 2

The Nafsiyat Intercultural Therapy Centre: Ideas and Experience in Intercultural Therapy

JAFAR KAREEM

It is now ten years since I attempted to define intercultural therapy as follows:

> A form of dynamic psychotherapy that takes into account the whole being of the patient – not only the individual concepts and constructs as presented to the therapist, but also the patient's communal life experience in the world – both past and present. The very fact of being from another culture involves both conscious and unconscious assumptions, both in the patient and in the therapist. I believe that for the successful outcome of therapy it is essential to address these conscious and unconscious assumptions from the beginning (Kareem, 1978).

The Nafsiyat intercultural therapy centre

The name Nafsiyat Centre arose out of the definition above: the word 'Nafsiyat' itself is composed of three different syllables, each coming from a different ancient language: they stand for MIND, BODY and SOUL (Kareem, 1987). This name was chosen to indicate that in this approach to patients we try to look at the whole person, as a social as well as a psychological being.

Nafsiyat was set up in London in 1983 to provide a specialist psychotherapy service to black and other ethnic and cultural minorities. Its work is concentrated in three main areas:

(1) *Clinical.* Nafsiyat offers therapeutic help to adults, families, adolescents and children who are experiencing psychiatric or sexual problems or emotional distress; it takes into account the racial and cultural component in mental illness.

(2) *Training and Consultation*. Training courses and seminars are organised in the field of intercultural therapy. Consultation on cases is given to other professionals in related fields.

(3) *Research*. Research is conducted into the efficacy of the treatment at Nafsiyat. New ways of therapy are developed through constant monitoring and evaluation of the work.

Referrals

Although the centre is based in North London, referrals come from all over London and also from other parts of the country. To date Nafsiyat has received about 2000 referrals from a variety of sources, including psychiatrists, general practitioners, social services and other mental health professionals. Interestingly, the largest group is comprised of those who refer themselves (see Chapter 6).

Ethnicity

We ask our patients to describe their own ethnic origin because we take a wide view of what constitutes 'ethnic identity'. Thus, for example, we have seen patients from France, Germany and South America. Allowing people to describe their ethnicity gives individuals the opportunity to describe themselves in the way they wish rather than being forced by us into a particular category. A young man born in Pakistan who came to this country at the age of five, for example, preferred to describe his ethnicity as 'Muslim' rather than as 'Pakistani' or 'Asian'. A woman born of Jamaican parents described her ethnic origin as 'African' but added, 'I have never been to Africa'. Our highest number of patients come from the African–Caribbean and South Asian populations, with most either born in Britain or growing up here. These are the people of whom it is said that they 'cannot respond to psychotherapy' (see also Chapter 1).

Therapy

Our approach to 'therapy' differs from that of many well established schools. The cause of an individual's distress is very difficult to define. It cannot be said that it is always a manifestation of the patient's inner psychic reality or part of his/her pathology as many orthodox schools in this field believe. In many cases, the overall responsibility for their distress may not lie with the patients at all. In our view socio-political and economic factors, over which the individual may have little or no control, affect the inner world of all of us. Our experience has led us not to accept that people from particular races have psychological insights whereas those from others have very few – a charge often levelled at people from African–Caribbean and Asian communities.

At Nafsiyat we aim to offer a form of dynamic psychotherapy which is not necessarily tied to one theoretical orientation but which derives its strength from various analytical, sociological and medical formulations. The object is to create a form of therapeutic relationship between the therapist and patient where both can explore each other's transference and assumptions. This process attempts to dilute the power relationship that inevitably exists between the 'help giver' and the 'help receiver'.

Our patients in therapy are allowed to choose their therapist and may, if they wish, bring an advocate with them into their sessions. They are also encouraged to negotiate such matters as the duration of therapy and times of appointments. Unlike some forms of therapy which encourage regression and dependency as a method of therapeutic encounter, our constant aim is to believe in the patients' ability to help themselves. Regular 'reporting back' by the patients, an integral part of our clinical work, allows them to feel that they have some control over what is happening in their own therapy. A detailed organisational account about how Nafsiyat functions has been given in two publications: the Nafsiyat Annual Report (for 1983) and 'Nafsiyat the First Five Years' (1989).

Some ideas in intercultural therapy

Any therapy which professes to ameliorate pain and to further healing must have some 'philosophical' and moral underpinning, a conceptual baseline from which therapists work. Psychotherapy is about human beings and therefore it must also be about humanity. A psychotherapeutic process that does not take into account the person's whole life experience, or that denies consideration of their race, culture, gender or social values, can only fragment that person. Similarly, we believe that racial difference between the therapist and the patient is counter-therapeutic when it is institutionalised in systems of power. One of the most important pillars of Nafsiyat's thinking is a belief in something we can call 'human universality': in practice, professionals should be able to work with all.

The idea of starting a specialist centre to offer psychotherapy to people from black and ethnic minority groups came out of my own experience of working as a psychotherapist in the National Health Service. Here, it became evident to me that patients from non-European societies were not responding to the type of psychotherapy they were being offered. It was both confusing and painful for me to come to terms with the fact that these patients from non-European societies appeared to be rejecting psychotherapy as it was practised at that time. This led me to question whether psychodynamically oriented psychotherapy is really suitable for non-white, non-European people (Chapter 12). At the same time there was a great deal of discussion about the 'inaccessibility' of psychotherapy to black and ethnic minority patients. We know that these patients were frequently only offered drug treatment and very rarely were given the option of having psychotherapy (Littlewood and Lipsedge, 1982).

It would be correct to say that such debates were the precursors to the formation of Nafsiyat in 1983. My own experience as an Indian, of living in a Western society and having been in analysis – a therapy of Western origin – brought out many conflicts in me, conflicts which I realised were not uncommon and which I hoped could be explored further for myself and others in a specialist clinical setting.

Experiences in intercultural therapy

It may be useful here to describe a case, the case of Victoria, which raises many of the key issues in intercultural therapy. I hope this will not so much show the psychotherapeutic processes at work but rather indicate the problems facing a member of an ethnic minority who is seeking appropriate help. The case illustrates the importance of colour and the experience of a 'Western' black person. I hope it also serves to illustrate the relationship between race and powerlessness, and how this can be an overriding factor in therapeutic work, as well as the importance of finding an identity that is linked to one's roots.

Case study

Victoria is now 26 years old. She was born in the United Kingdom and her family came from the West Indies. Her great grandparents were of different races, African and Spanish. Both sets of grandparents settled in the USA and her parents, both of whom were professionals, migrated to Britain. Victoria herself went to an expensive and well known private boarding school in England.

Because of Victoria's background – her English education and her cosmopolitan parents – one might have expected her to adjust easily to British society, and certainly not to require the services of a psychotherapist or that of a specialist minority organisation such as Nafsiyat. Victoria, however, had encountered quite a lot of overt racial hostility at her school. As she put it, 'You see, even so many years after the war, the English have never forgotten or forgiven what happened then. They still hate the Germans'. She went on, 'And, you know, some white people want blacks to forget all about slavery and colonisation. Whenever you mention it they say, "Oh, that's all in the past". Yes, there is no slavery now, and colonisation may not be flourishing, but we are still sub-human in some people's minds'.

At university Victoria became preoccupied with her blackness and became increasingly angry with her parents for having put her in this invidious position. Becoming curious about her ancestry and anxious to find a meaningful identity, she travelled around the world – to America, Africa and the West Indies – seeking clues about her family origins. She finally traced her father's line back to a young African woman, sold as a slave, forced to have children by many white men: 'All these people are linked to one woman who was picked up from Africa when she was young and sold as a slave. She produced many sons by white men . . . . You see, paternity of her children was imposed on her. Like many women, even now, she had no choice as to who fathered her children'. The unravelling of Victoria's history had a devastating effect on her. She became depressed and feared she was going 'mad'.

She then consulted a white woman therapist. But she found the therapist quite unable to give her the help she needed. 'The therapist made me feel that issues of race were essentially my problem. Whenever I tried to bring up anything relating to my feelings about being black, she always interpreted that as a projection of my inner chaos into the outside world. I felt angry and misunderstood. My pain and confusion was about being in a black/white situation where I was made to feel powerless.' In seeking help from Nafsiyat, Victoria said, 'I want a therapist who can immediately recognise my pain in being powerless and black in a society which is racist, and I want someone who can also work with my inner self'. The problem with the first therapist was not that she was white, but that she was unable to look at the inter-related themes of race and powerlessness as problems of reality.

Concepts of psychotherapy

European versus non-European

It has generally been acknowledged that psychodynamic psychotherapy was a European development, practised in Europe for European patients. It was taken for granted that the idea of a one-to-one relationship between patient and therapist was essentially unproblematic within European culture (Chapter 3). Can non-Europeans benefit from such a practice?

The cultural divergence between European and non-European societies is not confined to certain concepts of distress, dysphoria, or mental illness. There are radical differences in terms of day-to-day life, notions of the family and the role of its individuals, in child rearing, and ideas of education. There are also radical differences in 'cultural' attributes such as concepts of personhood, respect or disrespect, loyalty, independence, position of elders in the family, obligations to family and community – the very notions of moral tradition that combine to make a human being a social being rather than an isolated organism. An understanding of these aspects of human life is fundamental to the success of any therapy. What, then, does it mean to communicate across cultures? Is it possible at all to relate to a person with a totally different life experience? How do we make a bridge and attempt to comprehend the other person's experience? During the period of my own analysis, the free associations which came up included events, feelings and personal traumas which sometimes appeared totally meaningless – or even alien – to my therapist. At the beginning of the analysis assumptions were made and interpretations were given which took little account of who I was, where I had come from, or the nature of my early childhood upbringing. It may be difficult but it is surely not impossible for an analyst who has never had any experience of alternative life patterns to engage in a therapeutic relationship with a patient from a different race/culture. It certainly demands a great deal of effort on the part of the analyst to gather sufficient knowledge of the patient's culture. The need for psychotherapists to take such matters into consideration in both their practice and training is now acknowledged and this is evidenced in the proposals on intercultural therapy made by the United Kingdom Standing Conference for Psychotherapy.

To accept as part of the therapeutic model the working out of different cultural patterns in the human psyche brings to the forefront a vital question: how far can any human life experience be generalised? Can there be any sort of universal psychology? Beyond the fact of our shared humanity, individuals are unique and distinct from each other and thus there is always an interpersonal and 'intercultural' dimension to any encounter between two people, including that between therapist and client.

The concept of intercultural therapy

The Nafsiyat concept of intercultural therapy was developed from certain core ideas: that there are indeed some intrinsic differences between individual human beings, either in their biology, their personality or both, and that both inter- and intrapsychic events profoundly affect an individual's psyche and develop as part of their unconscious life. The events of the external world, then, are real but they are also internalised. Social and political phenomena are powerful forces, able to apply pressures not just on an autonomous person but determining the lives of individuals who live in a particular society.

In accepting and working with differences in human beings, however, one must try to seek the very universality that exists in diversity. Difference itself is universal, shared. In order to strive towards that goal it is accepted in the Nafsiyat model that external social factors such as prejudice, racism, sexism, poverty and social disadvantage – all of which cause profound pain, perhaps most especially for black and ethnic minority patients because of the situation they find themselves in – are real and must be taken into account as vital clinical concerns. They are part of the person. We are after all constituted by our pains as well as by our pleasures. The problem of having to constantly work through these originally external factors, as well as the individual's internal conflicts through which they may be represented, form the core of intercultural therapeutic work. Although Nafsiyat is a centre which is especially accessible for black and ethnic minority patients, we do not believe in separate services for any particular group. With such seeming contradictions in our own ideology, how then do we work with them in psychotherapy?

The historical context in therapy

If psychodynamic processes should take us back into the history of our ancestors – into the life experiences of our ancient loved ones; into the days of slavery, colonialism or other oppression – what emotions do these now generate in us when we meet someone whom we feel (in our fantasy) might have taken an oppressive role in that historical past? Is not that painful past history transmitted to us by each generation? Are we not constantly reminded by society that we may once have been slaves, once part of conquered nations or imperial rule? What impact might the constant reminder that someone is an outsider have on their psyche? It is impossible to determine how much the memory of the painful past forms part of our unconscious now, and how we react in a healing relationship with a person whom, unconsciously, we associate with that past.

Can we for a moment speculate upon what happens to analysts who have been brought up with the belief that some human beings are 'lesser than' other human beings? What in turn happens when they meet a patient who for a long time has considered *himself* to be less than a human being? Searching for answers to such questions is not easy. When I worked in Israel I often used to ask my Jewish friends and colleagues if they would agree to be in therapy with a non-Jewish German. Even amongst the most liberal the reply was always the same, 'the question could not arise, for a German who is not Jewish must have been associated with the Nazis'. Deep-seated feelings and rational everyday thinking do not always go hand in hand.

A mistrust of psychotherapy and its practitioners, not dissimilar to the above, prevails among many black and other minority groups in Britain. This situation seems to have come about due to the following:

(1) In spite of the fact that psychotherapy is available as one form of treatment, it is seldom offered to ethnic minority patients and even when it *is* offered it is rarely taken up (Littlewood and Cross, 1980; Moorhouse, Acharyya *et al.*, 1989; Campling, 1990).
(2) Many of the patients (a quarter of those seen in 1988) who referred themselves to Nafsiyat were black British: they had been born, brought up and educated in the UK but they happen not to have used and did not wish to use any other organisation offering psychotherapy (Moorhouse, Acharyya *et al.*, 1989).

Working with difference

The acknowledgement of diversity in human beings is an integral part of Nafsiyat's philosophy in as much as we believe that diversity brings life, vibrancy and (literally) colour to human society. Diversity and difference sometimes can, however, create tension and mistrust and this is an issue for all humankind. All we can try to do is to accept that any form of social power that is based solely on difference, of race, colour of skin, gender, religion or social and political affiliations, is anti-humanity and in the widest sense anti-sanity.

Clinical practice

Short-term therapy

As time went by, the workers at Nafsiyat gradually began to recognise that the centre would have to evolve a way of offering short-term dynamic psychotherapy. This was due to two important constraints:

- most of our patients responded better to short-term rather than long-term commitment;
- financial constraints on the organisation itself and lack of adequate staffing.

Although these two factors emerged independently, they enabled us to define a need and to formulate the option of offering short-term therapy. Since then our evaluation and research programme has established clearly that such therapy can be very effective (Chapter 6).

It should be added, however, that offering short-term therapy had, and still has, certain problems. As very few analytical therapists are trained to work on a short-term basis, it has on occasion been difficult to convince them that such therapy can be effective. Psychotherapists who have themselves been in long-term psychoanalysis or analytical psychotherapy, have found it painful not to be able to offer the same process to their patients. Some have the firm belief that all patients should receive long-term psychotherapy – for such people, it is the only acceptable way of working. Some therapists, confronted with the task of taking on patients at Nafsiyat, find it difficult, even from the beginning of therapy, to recognise that they are going to see a patient for short-term therapy that consists of only 12 sessions.

Having to deal with a frequent changeover of patients as well as the uncertainty of emotional and financial issues that are involved in short-term therapy, undoubtedly makes it difficult for a therapist to choose to work on a short-term basis – in spite of the fact that sometimes it may be beneficial to the patient. This fact has made it hard for all of us to re-orientate ourselves but we are learning all the time and we recognise that short-term therapy has many positive aspects and that it has been beneficial to a large number of our patients (Moorhouse, *et al.*, 1989).

Societal transference

The primary tools of psychotherapy are the interpretation of transference and working with the resulting countertransference. However, transference and countertransference occur not just as something that happens in the course of the therapeutic encounter itself: both patient and therapist, throughout their lives, carry inner feelings about others and these feelings become accentuated in the therapeutic situation. Inevitably, there occurs a social and communal transference related to other individuals and other groups of people and this plays an important role in the encounter even for experienced analysts. Such feelings lie in a very primitive part of ourselves. It should be recognised that a coloured person, because of his historical experience of discrimination, may carry a strong feeling generally about the white population – and that he may voice this in terms of their being hypocritical, insincere, complacent. Similarly, a white person will have, over the years, imbibed reciprocal feelings and notions about coloured people – as unsophisticated, emotional, or with a 'chip on the shoulder'.

In the transference situation, where we are dealing with the unconscious where both the patient and (let us admit) the therapist are vulnerable, these feelings come out into the open. What kind of transference takes place and what is the therapist able to do with it? How does the therapist deal with the patient's 'negative' transference as well as acknowledging his own negative counter-transference? We could, of course, speculate about which triggered off which. Nevertheless, for the therapist, the problem remains. Should they say, 'I think I know how you feel about me because you may have every reason to have strong feelings about who I represent to you?' Or, to a Jewish patient, something like, 'I am German and I did live in Germany during the last war'. Whose responsibility is it to bring these matters up in the therapeutic situation?

From the point of view of the intercultural therapist, I believe that it is the responsibility of the therapist, from the very outset, to facilitate the expression of any negative transference which is based on historical context, and not leave the onus on the patient. The patient may be too needy or too afraid and thus may not recognise the existence of negative feelings or may not consider them to be an immediate issue – indeed, he may consider them to be something perhaps to be denied in attempting a 'good relationship'. For the therapist who is working with a patient of a different background, however, it is a fundamental clinical issue which must be acknowledged and brought out into the open. This may be a difficult task but it is one that must be undertaken in order to facilitate therapy.

In understanding the history of European colonisation as well as the current social and political climate, it is perhaps not too surprising that patients from black and other ethnic minority groups are somewhat distrustful of white 'professionals'. And for all such professionals, the possibility of this mistrust needs to be allowed for from the very beginning. Neither patient nor therapist are 'innocent' of history and of memory. It is necessary to take into account that the relationship that currently exists between black and white people in our society will be mirrored in the therapist – patient relationship. If (and this is our experience at Nafsiyat) most black patients feel that they are devalued and dehumanised for 23 hours a day it is perhaps too much to expect them to feel anything different in the course of a one-hour session.

Intercultural matching of patient and therapist

I am aware that, put like this, the situation sounds rather depressing. It should not be concluded, however, that the patient should invariably be matched with a therapist from the same racial and cultural group. This is not necessary and is certainly not done at Nafsiyat. Indeed, here, a number of Europeans, including white English therapists, work with black and other ethnic minority patients. They learn to work cross-culturally and to constantly examine their practice as a part of a dynamic and growing process.

There is a great need for more working psychotherapists, indeed more professionals in all fields, from black and ethnic minority groups. They should not, however, be deployed to work exclusively with people from their own cultural group. Matching done purely on the basis of race or colour can imprison both the professional and the client in their own racial and cultural identity. It also diminishes the human element which must be an integral part of all professional encounters. Psychotherapists who are caught up in their own particular rituals always make heavy demands on their patients and tend to maintain them in a powerless situation. In such cases, the terms for therapeutic transactions are set by therapists and patients have little say in the matter (Limentani, 1986).

Power in psychotherapeutic alliance

It is noticeable that there is a great deal of hostility towards psychotherapy among minority groups because it is seen essentially as a 'Western, middle-class' form of treatment. White psychotherapists reciprocate by arguing that minority groups are not suitable for psychotherapy. This dynamic of suspicion is maintained from both sides, mirrored and double-edged. One of the major reasons for the distrust expressed by black patients is the inevitable imbalance of power that exists between therapist and patient. There is, of course, always a relationship of power implied when somebody comes to seek help from another and that other person gives that help. The receiver of help tends to feel vulnerable and powerless and as black and ethnic minority patients experience themselves as powerless in other situations they do not want this same situation to operate in a therapeutic encounter. This experience of powerlessness, especially for black patients, is a potent element in the therapeutic situation and one that must be addressed before work can start.

Another important power imbalance between therapist and patient is that of finance. Psychotherapists find it hard to accept that there is an inherent conflict of interest between therapist and patient when a financial transaction is a part of the treatment process. It is natural for the patient initially to want to progress sooner rather than later, not only because they wish to feel better, but also because they do not wish to go on incurring expense. Conversely, it may not be in the interest of therapists for patients to get better quickly if it means a decrease in their income – especially if those therapists are totally dependent on income from patients. The anxiety of losing a patient, and thus losing a part of one's livelihood, can have a devastating effect on the transference situation in therapy. Therapists need to be constantly aware of this lest financial pressures turn them into scavengers, always looking out for damaged (but not too damaged) people in order to maintain a satisfactory flow of patients. We cannot escape from the fact that our profession and livelihood depend on the availability of distressed human beings. It says something about the profession that, even now, most training in psychotherapy is in private hands and therapists are trained to work mainly in the private sector. Thus, high training fees act as a kind of exclusion clause as well as committing the training and trained therapists themselves to private work.

Profession or vocation?

Perhaps the practice of psychotherapy should ideally be a vocation rather than a profession. This does not mean, however, that practising psychotherapists should not be paid for their work, although it is helpful if they can have a secondary and independent source of income. Financial independence of therapists can be very liberating both for the patient and the therapist. It is my belief that, ideally, psychotherapists should be employed by public agencies or similar institutions and offer patients a free service. Nafsiyat (funded by Bloomsbury Health Authority and Islington Council) has operated such a service since its inception: the overwhelming majority of Nafsiyat's patients are from low income groups (Chapter 6).

Racism and therapy

As therapists at the Nafsiyat Centre primarily see patients from black and ethnic minority groups, working with racism both on inter- and intrapsychic levels forms one of the important aspects of our work. The concept of racism is in one aspect a psychological phenomenon; it affects whoever are its victims as well as its perpetrators. Since it is a reality of life for many people all over the world, including black people living in Britain, it is not helpful for us to explain it away simply as part of some people's psychic problem. But if its ultimate rationale is that of social power, racism, a two-way process, operates through primitive feelings of envy, hate, jealousy, greed, anger, violence, suspicion and fear. Most psychotherapists are supposed to have learned how to deal with these feelings, and yet most psychotherapists maintain that racism is not an issue for them, simply because it is a political (and thus 'external') issue. However, psychotherapists have been known to take a stand on the question of nuclear arms and other political issues (a welcome move indeed), but somehow or other they have failed to tackle or perhaps they shut their eyes to the racial issues which affect many people on their own doorstep. This may be because talking about and dealing with racial issues raises very painful emotions and touches everyone individually at some level.

I believe racism is not simply a black or a white problem. It is a human problem and one which includes all human beings and as such the struggle against racism cannot be separated from other struggles for human dignity and individual freedom.

Most psychotherapists who are analytically trained learn to work with and understand the patient's inner world only, and therefore for some there is resistance in dealing with psychological problems that originate in the real (outer) world. However, most black people would admit that the most traumatic feature in their personal lives is to be black in a white society. As Joseph, one of my patients, put it, 'We have been deprived of one of God's most precious gifts, the ability to "get lost", the ability to be anonymous, the ability not to be noticed. You cannot share the depth of this feeling with anyone, especially if you are constantly reminded that you are an outsider, that you and your like are swamping this country, that always you have to pass a test. What can you do?'

This particular patient had been in therapy elsewhere before he approached Nafsiyat. When I asked him if he had spoken about this sense of desolation with his previous therapist (who was white), he replied that he had not because there was no point. He admitted that he had been helped by the white therapist in many ways but still there was no 'meeting of the souls', as he put it, and he felt (rightly or wrongly) he could not bring up the issue of racism with his therapist.

Thus, even in an otherwise good therapeutic relationship, the therapist and the patient can operate on two parallel levels that reflect not only their own belief systems but their respective positions in society. We know that no patient can ever say everything no matter who the therapist. Both patient and therapist operate on the material, limited or not, that is produced in the course of therapy sessions. But an experience of such magnitude which generates such strong feelings cannot be left out if the therapy is to make any serious progress at all. It is a constant challenge for intercultural therapists to work with these inner and outer worlds simultaneously.

It is not very difficult to understand the problems of the white therapist who finds it hard to accept the experience of racism as a clinical matter. Painful descriptions of racial discrimination are often received with incredulity by white professionals because it is somehow extremely difficult for them to admit or accept that racial discrimination 'still exists'. One white therapist, explaining this to me in a private conversation, said, 'You know why? Because it never happens to us and it is beyond the realm of our inner or outer experience and hence we can easily deny it'.

Let me illustrate this point with a case history. This case shows how potentially damaging it can be to a patient if their real life experiences are not acknowledged in psychotherapy. These can be black/white issues, class issues or gender issues. In this particular case, the denial by the psychotherapist of the pain in the life experience of the black person brought the therapy process to an abrupt end.

Case study

I received a phone call from a colleague of mine who asked me whether I could help with his neighbour's son, John. He described the neighbours as a West Indian family who had experienced considerable difficulties in establishing themselves in this country. The father had abandoned the family when the children were very young and the mother had had to struggle very hard, first working as a cleaner in a hospital and then as a nurse. The son, John, was very intelligent, upright, slightly shy, and rather withdrawn. John had suddenly stopped going to his college classes or meeting friends socially and had locked himself up in his room. His mother had not been able to talk to him and she had now asked for my colleague's help.

John came to see me. He was brought by his step-father but I suggested I see John alone. He was a good-looking young man, a little nervous and solemn. I let him be for a few minutes and then told him how I had got involved and asked him if he wanted to say anything to me. He kept quiet for some time then mumbled something which sounded like, 'You won't understand' and I replied, 'Of course I won't understand if you do not want to say anything to me. But since you are here, it may be worth our while just to explore and find out whether I can understand you. Maybe I will, and maybe I won't.' John fidgeted in his chair, asked my permission to smoke and when I nodded, lit his cigarette, inhaled deeply, and looked at me steadily for a few seconds; then he told me this story.

He had always been a lonely person and mixed with a few select friends. During the final year of his studies one of his tutors had suggested that he should 'see somebody' to talk things over as the tutor had felt he was tense and did not appear to be concentrating, possibly because of lack of sleep. John had agreed because there were a lot of things on his mind – problems between his parents, his sister's unexpected pregnancy, his parents' reaction to this, the demands of his studies, and the pressures of his family on him to do well for he was considered the brightest in the family. Through his college he was referred to a psychotherapist whom he saw once a week during college hours. He did well in his final exams and got a good job. As he was now earning and was able to pay, he increased his therapy sessions to twice a week. Because of his work commitments his appointments with his therapist took place early in the morning.

At this point he became quiet again and looked vacantly into space. After some time I commented, 'And so?' John looked at me, turned away his face and with a lot of anger suddenly said, 'This is what happened . . . . One dark winter morning I was waiting at a bus stop to go to see my therapist. There were one or two people in the queue and as the bus was late in coming I was feeling very anxious. I started to fidget in my pocket looking for my bus-pass. Suddenly a police car drew up and two policemen jumped out of the car and made me stand against a wall. They searched me all over. I was very angry and frightened and did not know what was happening to me. When I questioned the policemen, one of them said I was behaving suspiciously and they wanted to check me out because they thought I had drugs on me. When

I said I had a doctor's appointment and produced my student card to show I was educated, the policeman laughed at me saying, "Oh no, you're not going to college. You are coming with us".

I was absolutely staggered and in a rash moment suggested to the policemen that they should follow me. They both burst out laughing and one of them actually got into the bus with me and the other followed in the car. They were having a good joke at my expense. In the bus I was sweating and I was wet all over although it was a cold morning. When I actually arrived at the therapist's door and rang the bell, the policemen were still laughing at me. However, my therapist came out and took me in. I was too overwhelmed and shocked and could not speak during my session. My therapist kept quiet and the silence infuriated me and at one point I could not hold myself back and blurted out in an angry voice something like,"You don't understand". By this time I was crying but still my therapist said nothing and I could no longer contain myself and told my therapist what had happened to me on my way there. There was a silence I could not bear. Then my therapist said to me, "You are expressing this anger because I am white". I was stunned because until that moment it had not mattered to me that the therapist was white. And then when my therapist added "I never thought you were black, I just took you to be another human being", I could bear it no longer and I left my session.'

John told me that after that episode he lost his faith that he was a human being and became frightened to go out. Whenever he walks on the street and sees an old lady crossing the road clutching her handbag, he involuntarily stops and asks himself, 'Do I look like a mugger?' He said it often takes him a few minutes to get over this feeling.

John suddenly got up from his chair and started pacing furiously up and down my room; his fists were clenched and his face contorted as if he was going to explode – and he did: he screamed, 'I hate you all. I hate my parents for giving birth to me. I hate being black. Most of all I hate being imprisoned by my black skin'.

Whenever I have mentioned such cases to groups of psychotherapists or social workers they sometimes react with over-enthusiastic interest as if I am presenting some exotic material, or else with deadly silence as if I am trying to provoke guilt in white professionals, and sometimes with remarks like, 'yes, I know that, but it is not only black people who suffer; as a white person I also feel afraid to go to Brixton at night'. Such comments are made quite often and once a black person in the group was moved to respond in these words, 'You are afraid to go to Brixton. I am afraid to go anywhere'.

Incidents of racial harassment of black people in our society abound (Commission for Racial Equality, 1990; Rose and Liston, 1990). I am not implying here that the blame lies simply with the white population or with white professionals or that in some way because of them black people suffer from mental illness. I do not believe in a conspiratorial theory in which white psychiatrists and other professionals deliberately misdiagnose, mistreat or misjudge black and other ethnic minority patients. As in any society, there are professionals who may harbour conscious or unconscious racist attitudes but I am also equally aware that there are many white professionals who are constantly fighting racism wherever they find it, in or out of health services, and who are fully aware of the extent of the problem.

The sense of loss

The concept of loss of a very early love object and subsequent manoeuvres to cope with such loss, constitute, according to some, the basis for many later emotional traumas. In Western society, where the concept of a single set of biological parents is deeply embedded in normative assumptions, the loss of a parental figure, especially the mother who feeds the infant, is considered to be of immense significance.

Is this concept of loss of attachment to a parent figure universal, however? In a non-Western culture where there are 'multiple parents', surrogate mothers and fathers and other relations who undertake a great deal of mothering and fathering of children, how is the sense of loss experienced? Talking to many patients, from many different cultures, who have been reared and cared for by grandparents, uncles and aunts in an extended family, one comes to recognise that their sense of loss encompasses a much wider dimension than one where there is just one individual parent. They talk of their loss in terms of multiple relations, in terms of the loss of their roots, of their society, of their environment, and of memories of multiple caring adults. How does one deal with such a sense of widespread loss when one has little comprehension of it?

Individuals are influenced and affected by their early experiences of childhood; and in a society where bonding between a child and its biological mother or nuclear parents is considered the norm, it is not uncommon for many white professionals to find it difficult to understand the implications of the family patterns in African and West Indian families. In their bewilderment it is also not uncommon for such therapists to make comments such as: 'This child must have been damaged by the multiple relationships of the mother or father. There is little I can do', or, 'Brought up by grandparents – why? What were the parents doing? If the children have joined their parents here [in the UK] at such a late stage what can you expect but very disturbed behaviour?'

If professionals in the UK remain set in their belief that what matters most is encompassed in their own idea of family and child-rearing, then other mothers and carers with their own ideas are placed in an inferior position. I remember an occasion outside the UK when an African man had come to see me – he was a highly educated and intelligent man working as an expert for an international agency. He consulted me about a minor emotional problem and during the course of my discussions with him, he revealed to me with great joy and emotion, that he was loved and cared for by thirteen different mothers, his father's wives and partners, and said with much warmth, 'It was not just one pair of hands or one pair of breasts that continuously fed me, cuddled me and cared for me. I was a prince among princes'. In a Western family setting this would appear abnormal, indeed 'damaging'.

Training in psychotherapy

There is no obligation on a particular psychotherapist to work with patients who belong to different social or cultural groups. Most psychotherapists can choose who they work with. Working with people who are different can impose certain strains on the therapist. To take on a patient from a vastly different racial and cultural group, where there may be major differences in basic human concepts and values, can be both demanding and challenging – the likelihood of failure in such a situation seems inherent. Few psychotherapists or psychotherapy training organisations are prepared to take up the intercultural challenge. Their defence is that they treat all human beings as the same, even if society at large may not yet do so.

Can psychotherapists have a moral sense of duty to other human beings as individuals without having a parallel obligation to them as members of society? Do they – or should they – have some accountability to the community at large and to their role within it? Can they be totally immune from the forces that operate in society and ignore the world in which they live? Can they escape into their consulting rooms with no one to whom they are accountable?

As has been said, as far as psychotherapy training programmes in this country are concerned, not many training organisations have yet taken up the intercultural issues outlined in this book. Many candidates from black and other minority groups admit to finding most training programmes sterile and unmeaningful. They feel inhibited about openly bringing up issues of racism either in their analysis or within their training organisations. Many feel the pressure to keep quiet to be immense, the pressure to finish their training, to get the piece of paper which enables them to earn a living. In the light of the above, people who are totally dependent on patients for their livelihood dare not, especially if they are black, express views which are not acceptable. The rigid compliance demanded by some training organisations can also be contrary to the personal and professional growth of psychotherapists and the healthy development of the profession. It is interesting (and encouraging) to note that many psychotherapy training organisations are now engaged in debate on this matter.

It is, of course, debatable whether psychotherapeutic training that is wholly tied to the European model of mind and its psychological concepts is any longer able to meet the task of today's mobile and pluralistic society (Kakar, 1985). Training in psychotherapy needs to take a universal view of the human psyche and of human suffering – to encompass religious values as well as psychological complexes.

It is interesting to note that during the last few years many white psychotherapists have expressed an interest in working with black patients and there are signs that some training organisations are beginning to take steps to attract black trainees into psychotherapy. However, this has been, and still is, a very difficult process. On the one hand, many psychotherapists wish to take a 'colour-blind' approach; on the other hand, some feel that taking these issues into consideration may in itself appear discriminatory, however 'positively' so. While 'positive discrimination' may seem to be a negative step, not taking into account a person's race at all denies part of the basic essence of that person and may create the impression that there is an unconscious wish that one day everyone will be 'the same'. This view ignores the fact that a black person, however Westernised, will always be seen as a black person. Indeed, this whole process reflects the difficulty that all of humankind have in dealing with and accepting difference and diversity.

Perhaps at this point the reader will forgive a personal reminiscence about my own training and experience of analysis. During the time I was developing the concepts of intercultural therapy, I found that one of the most difficult things was for me to look deep into myself and to realise from what point I was starting and where I was, and to re-examine how much my analysis, my training process, and the process of acquiring a new skill had affected me. My own internal ego and superego had become replaced with the external institutional superegos of my training models. It was very difficult to break away from these models since they had become, not only part of my inner self and my external gestures and manners, but could well have taken me over completely.

Such intensive training can sometimes be compared to a kind of colonisation of the mind and I constantly had to battle within myself to keep my head above water, to remind myself at every point who I was and what I was. It was a painful and difficult battle not to think what I had been told to think, not to be what I had been told to be and not to challenge what I had been told could not be challenged and at the same time not to become alienated from my basic roots and my basic self. It had not been easy in the first place to reject many things that were part of me from the day I was born in order to replace them with some very sophisticated new ideas and techniques. My authenticity was almost lost in favour of this 'new know-ledge'. For me, the process of re-evaluation was cataclysmic because it demanded that I step outside my immediate (and convincing) new frame in order to question the relevance of what I was learning. Liberating ourselves from our masters, teachers, analysts and institutions is one of the most difficult tasks but without such a breaking free not much in the way of personal development can take place.

It is not possible to produce some kind of ten-point programme of skills in the field of intercultural therapy that one can learn. Nor do we attempt to do this in this book. In working with patients from different racial and cultural groups, much will depend on the individual therapist's acumen, their openness and awareness of the issues involved.

As most of the black and other ethnic peoples who have settled in the UK and other Western countries have come from areas which were once under colonial power, psychotherapy cannot be expected to operate and be meaningful without taking into consideration the effects of colonial rule on these individuals. In a psychotherapeutic situation after all one needs to understand the processes of power and how they operate. Sometimes they are a matter of straightforward coercion and subjugation, but at other times more subtle and insidious but no less brutal (see Chapter 12).

This chapter does not attempt a political analysis of the effects of colonialism, nor is it an attempt to lay blame on colonialism for all the damaging social and economic aspects of the colonised country's politics and society. As a person born in India, I am very aware that India was a fragmented society even before colonial rule and that social injustice and prejudicial practice based on religion, economic status, caste and sometimes on colour were prevalent in India, and still are. However, the occupation of another nation by military force does change the dimension of human relationships. Any relationship based on the total power of one group, whether between nation and nation, community and community, individual and individual, where one group is totally subjected to the power of the other, is both demeaning and destructive to both sides; in effect it destroys humanity.

How and why small but powerful occupying forces all over the world are able to take over vast countries, huge sections of humanity, to enslave them or impose the values of the occupying power is a very large question indeed. How was it possible for Britain to colonise India, for example, a much older civilisation, and to undermine the value systems which had existed there for generations? It seems to me that in this situation psychological occupation was much more damaging and long-lasting than physical occupation. It destroyed the inner self. All occupying forces strive to find people in the occupied territories whose minds can be colonised, so that the colonisation process can be continued through them, through thoughts rather than physical coercion. This process has a long-lasting effect which can continue through generations after colonisation has ended (Mannoni, 1964).

The very few black therapists who have gone through the process of analysis know well the struggle that has to be faced. In order to survive one complies, and sometimes, unconsciously, one becomes the other, the coloniser; one becomes, or pretends to become, what one is not. However, this dilemma can be understood in terms of the insidiousness of the psychological, social and, perhaps most importantly, the economic power that has operated. People in this position want to appear 'respectable' and to conform. After all, you earn your living from private patients and if you want patients to be referred to you, you must adhere to the rules of the club (whether white *or* black). Therapists from such ethnic backgrounds – and their teachers – are now becoming aware of the above processes and recognise the need to retrieve and reclaim their rich history and traditions, those either destroyed, buried, or forgotten under colonialism. Hence there is a great surge of parochial feeling among black professionals with its obvious inherent dangers. The way forward is for the present training institutions to take into account the racial and cultural dimension in the therapeutic process so that the whole training in psychotherapy does not become divisive and disintegrated.

Manifestations of mental illness

Illness or distress

There have been many debates about the incidence of mental illness among ethnic minorities and how it manifests in different cultures and races. For intercultural therapy it is necessary to understand how the patient him- or herself first experiences and perceives their illness or problem, in effect, to allow them authenticity as a person. It is therefore useful to involve patients themselves from the outset, to let them explain and define how they see their own problem whether in terms of bodily disease or emotional distress.

Intercultural therapy is not only a therapy where therapist and patient come from different races but also one where any kind of difference in culture is reflected in their attitudes and concepts of life, in their manifestations of distress and in their personal ideas about what might be done or can be done.

Problems in therapy where therapist and patient share the same background: the case of Mr Jagganath

The case below illustrates the diverse concepts of 'self' in a particular society,

Indian, where self is seen as a part of a multiple self. It explores the conflict of identity that this may create and also illustrates the notion of individuality in relation to family and community, the effect which family hierarchy can have on an individual, and the role of family and religious traditions in a changing society.

Case study

A middle-aged Indian man came to see me along with his hospital social worker. The social worker told me that she had become involved as the patient had been living alone and had withdrawn from all outside contacts. He had remained within his flat but appeared incapable of shopping or of even cooking his own food. He had asked for help and was given a home-help then refused to accept this so the Social Services Department felt there was no other option but to admit him to hospital.

When the patient entered my room I was struck by his appearance. He was a tall, fair, striking-looking man with long flowing hair down to his shoulders and a big red mark on his forehead. He carried a stick in his hand and as he entered my room he looked me over and stretched out his hand and told me, 'I am Maharaj Jagganath.' He added, 'You must be from Malaysia. I can speak to you in Malay if you like.' He then added, referring to the social worker, 'that will serve her right, as she will not understand anything'. I shook his hand and said to him that I did not speak any Malay and that I came from India. He was delighted and said, 'Now you will understand me and you will solve all my problems'. His expectations made me feel nervous and I became aware that he was certainly making some assumptions about me. I was also aware that he would expect me to side with him and it could be tempting for me to collude in this.

'Collusion' is defined as an inappropriate support for the patient's own wishes and it is a concept psychotherapists often talk about. Whenever I raise the point that it may on occasion be therapeutically beneficial (and I have to make this point clear) for a black patient to see a black therapist, the question of collusion is raised by white colleagues. This issue is one that is seldom mentioned and therefore is disregarded whenever white professionals work with white patients.

Early on in our session Mr Jagganath indicated that he wanted to speak to me on his own, so, as soon as the social worker had left us, he said to me, 'Let me make one thing clear – I am a Brahmin, I am a Punjabi, I am British and I am an Indian. I am all those four together and that is what I want you to write in your file. Whenever I speak, all those four speak from inside me. And as you see they (the social workers) have got a problem and they don't know what to do with me.' I asked him to elaborate and he explained that he was the eldest in a family of four brothers and two sisters. Recently his father, who was a well-known businessman, had died and now it had fallen on him to become the head of the household. Mr Jagganath had been in this country for the last twenty years and he had continued to live as a strict Brahmin, while his father and brothers and sisters had become Westernised.

On the death of his father, when Mr Jagganath became the head of the family, he wanted to change the way in which the family affairs were run. He wanted to introduce a strict Brahminical code of behaviour, ban alcohol, and introduce regular religious worship at home. However, his authority was challenged, first by his own youngest son, who was studying physics. He described this son as someone 'who has lost his head' and who was eating meat. This disobedience from his son had caused him immense anger and pain but when his own younger brothers and sisters sided with his son he said, 'Then there was nothing left for me to live for. I know my father had become a bit Westernised but deep down he was a good man and a good Brahmin and I am sure he would want me to help the family. Now I have let him down but most important of all I have let down my community and my religion. I decided that the time had come for me to give up everything.' He felt very strongly that his son's first commitment should be to him and to the family. 'We all must sacrifice ourselves for our beliefs, for our religion, for our family, otherwise what is the meaning of life?'

Although I come from India myself (albeit from a different tradition and region) this case presented me with a complex problem. As a psychotherapist I was aware of this patient's psychic process of projection and splitting. I also knew that I had to work within a context which was real and meaningful to him. This was represented in a conflict within myself as to whether I really wished to work with him or not. In the end I decided to take him on as he seemed to have made a good contact with me and expressed a definite wish to continue.

My relationship with Mr Jagganath and our sessions were problematic as he was always excessively polite and tried to use my 'Indian-ness' in a rather manipulative way. It was difficult for me to be very firm with him but he was, nevertheless, one of the (rare) patients at whom I shouted, and I even told him to leave my room on one occasion. Whenever I challenged him he would claim his superiority as a pure Aryan Brahmin and would try to put me down because I have a Muslim name. He would do this in a pained and sad voice and we would laugh hilariously together for we both understood that he was trying again to please me by pretending to be mortified. The fact that he kept coming to his sessions regularly (although unable to use public transport at the beginning) and made good progress, confirmed for me that it had been right to take him on. I had to work very hard with his transference and my own countertransference and to be constantly aware of this dynamic process in every session. By the time his course of treatment with me had ended he had moved back into his family home having first arranged for all his meals to be cooked separately by a Brahmin cook, and in general he seemed more reconciled to his family.

Reflections on therapeutic encounters

Patients' rights

Patients who seek psychotherapy have a right to know about the therapist's training and experience. In my view they should question their prospective therapists about this and whether they are fully trained or still in training and whether they are being supervised. It is possible for therapists to answer such questions without being defensive. Patients are also quite justified in enquiring about the professional affiliations of any therapists they are consulting. They should be encouraged to 'shop around' for a psychotherapist and I think this idea should be promoted by all organisations.

Trainee psychotherapists are understandably often 'coy' about disclosing the fact that they are trainees. Now that the psychotherapy profession is becoming organised under the United Kingdom Standing Conference for Psychotherapy, it is to be hoped that it will be possible for organisations to declare to prospective patients the true status of the therapist they are recommending. As we grow up and have more confidence in ourselves and in our profession, we will become secure enough to say who we are!

The relative powerlessness of the patient in the therapeutic situation needs to be recognised. Where possible the patient should be given a choice about the therapist and the right to negotiate about other aspects of therapy. This might suggest 'pleasing the patient' at all costs, responding to their pathological needs and avoiding their need to work through painful situations. However this has not been our experience at Nafsiyat. In contrast, having the opportunity to negotiate and have some say in their treatment plan seems to motivate our patients and enable them to engage in treatment.

At the Nafsiyat Centre I always start my first session with an acknowledgement that it must be very difficult for the patient to come and seek help from another person about whom he or she may know nothing. Similarly, if the patients, most of whom are black, tell me their life-story without telling me how it feels to be black in this society, I point out this omission and encourage the patient to explore why they have left out that particular bit of their life experience.

Reflecting on our experiences at Nafsiyat I feel that these steps, namely taking up the issue of negative transference and recognising patients' feeling of powerlessness, psychologically, politically and socially, were perhaps major breakthroughs in our relationships with our patients and contributed towards making the experience of coming to Nafsiyat relevant to so many of them.

This process has also allowed me to 'be myself' with my patients. For me, spontaneity and the freedom to *be* myself without the restraints of too many therapeutic rituals are essential ingredients in fostering the kind of 'authentic relationship' without which I believe no healing is possible. When patients ask me questions, especially about myself, I attempt, while trying to interpret their anxiety, to also answer their query as honestly as possible. Without dissolving the distinctions that necessarily exist between the patient and myself I can also let myself scream and shout if need be in my sessions – I have been known to scream a patient out of my room. Similarly I feel free to be sad and depressed and also to jump for joy with my patients. I would also say that for psychotherapists to question often and to doubt sometimes is the prerequisite for development and growth. For them. And for their patients.

Chapter 3

How Universal Is Something We Can Call 'Therapy'?

ROLAND LITTLEWOOD

Therapy: from Proto-Indo-European *ar* ('way of being, orderly and harmonious arrangement of the parts of a whole'), and thus Hittite *tarpan-alli* ('ritual substitute'). (After Tyler, 1986.)

Psychotherapy as a discipline is haunted by a question posed (especially) by psychiatrists and psychologists of an empirical turn of mind: 'Yes, but does it work?' There is now general agreement that whatever his original intentions were, the central theories of Freud's psychoanalysis are less some type of natural science hypothesis which can be experimentally verifiable in any context, than a general model of human personality and development, furthermore developed within the very specific cultural context of his own clinical work with patients. A common criticism of 'intercultural therapy' is that, not only has it too not yet been shown to be effective in ways we can measure objectively (but see Chapter 6), but that the application of psychotherapy outside the original European middle-class milieu is limited (Mullings, 1984). It is argued that all therapies – family therapy possibly excepted (see Maranhão, 1984 and Chapter 8, this volume) – start from certain shared but limited notions of what constitutes both 'problem' and 'therapy'. All therapy works in, and is constrained by, its own context; any evaluation can only make sense in that context and with those meanings.

Deleuze and Guattari (1984), in their attack on the primacy of the Oedipal pattern in theory and therapy, argue that the Oedipal triangle (father, mother, child) already exists as part of the modern bourgeoisie's self-conception. It is less an existing social structure than an ideology; thus therapies which claim to resolve problems arising in the Oedipal situation are not something technical which is applied from the outside but are themselves already part of the organisation and legitimation of the nuclear family's own 'myth' about itself. It is less therapy in fact than part of the sickness.

The British anti-psychiatrists of the 1960s 'Counterculture', Laing and Cooper, made a similar point but more pragmatically: they perceived severe psychopathologies as an identifiable state of being which could be examined and alleviated rather than as a figure of speech. But they too identified the contemporary 'Western family', or at least its ideal representation, as 'pathogenic' (Laing and Esterson, 1964; Cooper, 1971). I do not propose to debate here the legitimacy of their argument in the light of more recent studies on the cross-cultural epidemiology of severe mental illness and on its prognosis in relation to family response, but to start with this problem of distinguishing 'actual illness' from the social context and from the 'treatment' itself.

For example, is depression in people who regard themselves as racially oppressed, an 'abnormal' response? Can we argue that it has perhaps its own legitimacy, one perhaps that reflects social rather than therapeutic resistance? Is our emphasis on 'therapy' then a refusal to recognise or to acknowledge the political? How, in any case do we set about differentiating the 'therapeutic' from the 'political': by social context or by the language and metaphors which structure our experiences? Do we rely on people's own understandings or on a more detached analysis? We know that the language of psychopathology is already used to define social institutions that are seen as deviant or dysfunctional from the perspective of the speaker (Littlewood, 1984a; Gilman, 1985). The black American family is seen as a 'tangle of pathology'; the undesirable Third World politician as 'paranoid' (Bremner, 1991).

When we talk of psychological or behavioural difficulties where there is evidence of associated biological dysfunction which we interpret as causative – brain tumours, vitamin deficiencies, thyroid abnormalities – the language of biomedicine seems generally acceptable. We appear to have no difficulty here in making clear distinctions between *disease* (an underlying biological change), its representation as *illness* (our personal expression and response to disease), and the *therapy* which is offered to counter the underlying disease process and hence diminish illness[1]. When we consider problems where there is no obvious biological component, we seem here to apply the idiom of 'pathology' to a variety of institutional problems only because we live in a highly medicalised society in which distress is regarded as a purely individual phenomenon. It is difficult to clearly separate the 'problem' itself from those underlying cultural or political patterns which may be said to 'cause' it or, alternatively, of which we may argue it may be merely one manifestation (Littlewood, 1991).

Let us take two instances: that of *anorexia nervosa* and of deliberate overdose with prescribed drugs. Various critics of psychiatry have argued that anorexia is simply an extreme demonstration of women's 'expected' body shape in a political context where female morphology is determined by men, and where thinness confers certain social advantages. Overdoses, similarly, are only a logical extension of the medicalisation of women, as demonstrated, for example, in the advertisements in medical journals encouraging doctors to prescribe psychotropic (mind-influencing) medicines for depressed house-wives (Littlewood and Lipsedge, 1987). And yet, it is difficult to say we are simply dealing with a manifestation of male power, in which women are helpless victims and in which male preoccupations are inscribed on women's bodies by women themselves. For the subjective experience of such 'pathologies' is frequently one of attaining increased control over one's life. Are they then adaptive strategies of everyday resistance that are 'carried too far'? We can argue that even in the form in which they result in hospitalisation, the results may enhance individual autonomy and control. But at a cost. From the medical (and psychodynamic) perspective they remain maladaptive.

However we read such patterns, it is by no means obvious where 'pathology' is to be located: in the social structure, in the oppression of women, or in the individual's own subjectivity, self-identity or actions. The language of medicine – with its clear distinction between aetiology, pathology, symptoms and therapy – makes sense within our particular context. It makes sense to us, either as patients or therapists, because we are embedded in that particular context; as people who inhabit a particular shared world, we also share certain concepts and concerns. How could we not? I am not arguing for a therapy which is independent of these powerfully embedded social meanings – for could there be such a process when the very distinction between cause, pathology and therapy is in itself a social construct? I would suggest, however, that our distinction between, (a) the problem, and (b) its resolution, is one to be examined. Therapies and therapists of all types are part of the political field which includes the identified problem. We cannot presume that 'therapy' has the ultimate consequences which are explicitly sought. After all, the meanings and motivations which we ascribe to others may be quite different from those of the people concerned.

Other therapies, other problems

I have concentrated on the case of gender, in part because these points have been better argued already by the women's therapy movement in which the ambiguities of autonomy through pathology have become a therapeutic concern. Similar considerations apply to culture and to race. If, at one reading, therapy may be argued as resolving social antagonisms which, through our emphasis on medicalisation, only gain individual representation as a sickness, then, in the area of intercultural work, we must proceed with our eyes open. The obvious 'liberal' approach is one which simply seeks to offer the European therapeutic model to others on the basis that this is the best we have and that common justice invites us to extend its application. Unless the very problem for which we extend it is our very selves? Any 'radical' critique would argue precisely this: that the provision of 'white' therapies for 'black' people presenting with problems that result from existing patterns of white-black dominance is problematic, to say the least. At its strongest, this argument would seem to implicate psychotherapy as only a more insidious variant of European middle-class authority, denying to others even the authenticity of their own expression of distress: thus transforming and condensing down 'political' tensions into the less inconvenient form of 'individual' pathology.

Where does this leave the therapist? Liberally minded white professionals and their institutions remain compelled to act, whether by administrative power, external criticism or through a notion of common humanity which – in theory at least – encompasses us all.

At this point in the debate the question can only be argued in the abstract. Until different forms of therapy, either ethnically-matched or cross-cultural and cross-racial, have been attempted, we cannot argue either for or against some kind of 'black therapy'. This applies whether this is one which is political, unifying all black suffering under a rubric of oppression or resistance, or one which reaffirms some 'traditional' and uncontaminated form of 'therapy' (whether this is perceived by the sociological observer as religious, magical, pragmatic or other).

For the rest of this chapter I shall side-step this debate in order to look at some other therapeutic contexts, not those of 'pure' uncontaminated traditions (for these do not exist) but those of other patterns which recall European psychotherapy. To what extent can an argument be made for common features? What would such common features be: a theory of psychology resembling the European model; a procedure whose formal characteristics and personnel recall those of our Hampstead or hospital consulting rooms; a process of individual or group change which is amenable to a conventional psychodynamic explanation? Or, alternatively, some sort of structural relationship between ideology, individual and therapeutic process which is similar to those we can identify in the West?

We can certainly demarcate the useful limits of comparison. All societies make distinctions between desired and undesired states of being, and have standardised forms of reconstructing experience, through the response of other people, to return the individual back to a state desired by individual and community alike. At such a level of abstraction, 'therapy' is universal. We might note that the explicit construction of 'distress' – whether as sickness, pollution, possession, psychopathology or sorcery – varies considerably. At the level of external analysis, however, analogous patterns of underlying 'tensions' – generational and gender conflicts, intra- and intergroup relations – may be articulated through these widely differing explanations of what constitutes misfortune. 'Universality', if we happen to find it, will be in the head of the (usually European) observer, for no 'local' system of therapy, psychoanalysis excepted, makes a claim to interpret all the other systems.

By contrast, in a more restricted sense, psychotherapy is not universal. The theories of transactional or Kleinian analysis are hardly those to be found in other societies. While we can note similarities, we cannot 'translate' one set of understandings into another without a significant loss of meaning.

The illustrations of this that I offer will be derived mainly from accounts given by social anthropologists. While social anthropology, like psychother-apy, is a 'Western' academic discourse rooted in Western institutions of power and representation, I would argue that it does provide some more 'distanced' perspective in that its own, admittedly limited, comparative language of 'structure', 'dominance' and 'opposition' can also be applied with some value to Western institutions themselves. If we take specifically psychological constructs and states – 'unconscious', 'insight', 'ego-syntonic' – as the initial starting point, we assume in advance the procedures of Western psychology and the dominance of something like psychiatry to be 'therapy'. We shall return to these issues later.

Societies, it must be said, seem to get along quite well without a formal and elaborated system of 'psychology'. If the numbers of words we have available to describe moods and states of mind – our affective lexicon – is taken as the determining measure of our psychological life (as it has been by psychiatrists such as Leff (1981)), then cultures can proceed with remarkably few terms, in some cases less than ten (Howell, 1981). This does not mean that individual life and identity are not distinguished and selected out for remark, amplifica-tion or change, but that the world view itself is constructed rather differently. The so-called 'multiple souls' of West African systems of understanding (Prince, 1964) may be described as attributes of individual identity which can conflict with each other: some are derived from paternal kin, others are associated with natural forces, others are the expression of individual choice (Horton, 1983). It would be as inappropriate to translate them into the language of psychology (so that 'souls' became 'faculties', and our father-, nature- and choice-souls became the super-ego, id and ego of Freud's structural schema), as to do the reverse. The two systems are merely different ways of understanding how we as individuals are yet 'not' individuals. As distinct persons, we share characteristics with the natural world, with our kin and significant others, and yet we do not experience ourselves as completely determined from 'the outside'.

The primacy of psychology in the West is a relatively recent phenomenon.

And to identify as a universal experience all the connotations of 'depression' that are packed together as a discrete category, for example, is mistaken. While the physical symptoms of severe depression appear to have some universality, and a state akin to misery, dejection and self-doubt may be said to occur everywhere, the clinical and subjective experience of 'depression' (a phenomenological sinking downwards of the self) is hardly universal (Kleinman and Good, 1985). Indeed, Shweder (1985) argues that the experience of something being removed out of oneself, already well described in the Latin American experience of soul loss, *susto*, is even more common across the world.

Gender politics: a Kenyan example

The experience of *saka* (which we might describe for the moment as 'possession') was once not uncommon among the Waitata of Kenya (Harris, 1957). Half of the women in the community developed saka at some time during their lives. In a situation where women were expected not only to provide the food for their families, but also domestic utensils and household objects, they did not have access to the necessary money for these things since this was generated through the sale of land and livestock and these were the concern of men alone since women were said to have 'no head for land or cattle transactions'. Saka occurs when women are denied a request made to their husbands, typically for something which men consider their own prerogative.

The pattern of saka, which was described by Western observers as 'hysteria', provides a social caricature of women as uncontrollable consumers, as vulnerable, emotional and out of control. 'They are shown as contrasting in every way with men and the contrast is symbolised as a personal malady.' The therapy? The husband sponsors a large public ceremony in which his wife wears items of male dress or new clothes: this constitutes an inversion of normal behaviour which, from the outside, we might see as a 'resolution' of domestic conflict. Described baldly like this, saka seems a transparently adaptive device, hardly to be considered an illness. From the local perspective, at least from that of the men, saka may indeed be understood as an illness but also as the undesirable attack of malign spirits, and as the simple expression of women's social position and 'personality'. Nor do we find that all the men in the society always see the reaction in the same way. All patterns of distress and misfortune are flexible, sometimes tentatively performed, sometimes hinted at, and they exist not just through discrete and dramatic patterns like saka but as part of everyday conversations and conflict.

If my brief account serves to make the pattern transparently 'adaptive' for individual women, local men would argue that the whole thing may be simulated. Its 'otherworldly' power nevertheless compels the community to action through the obligations inherent in 'illness' or 'possession'. We might remark on the parallels with overdoses in Britain. Both the woman who takes the overdose, and her family and the medical staff in the casualty department, make distinctions between the overdose as the 'symptomatic' expression of an underlying despair or as a transparently instrumental 'manipulative' action. To what extent are the psychological experiences in overdoses and saka identical? The answer lies, not in some state abstracted from context, deprived of social meaning, but in the sort of 'fit' with available models which we may identify, if we choose, with isolation and despair or even rebellion. To note the social consequences is not to label the protagonist/patient as a callous actor, but to affirm the cultural meaning of suffering of any type. If the whole pattern (context, precipitating episode, 'symptoms', resolution) may be said to 'work' for the individual and her community, then it only works through the power which compels us to respond to the threat of illness or possession. Nor can we argue that the pattern is always 'adaptive'. Saka, like the overdose, may at times be ridiculed or ignored, or indeed become part of a continuing pattern not easily seen as 'adaptive' for the individual woman herself.

Gender politics: a Somalian example

A similar pattern, *sar*, occurs among the nomadic Somali. Here, the possessing power is clearly identified as female itself, jealous of men's authority (Lewis, 1966). Women are normally excluded from public decision making and power, except in the resolution of sar. The members of the community who are accepted as able to recognise and treat sar attacks are people who have previously been victims themselves; indeed, they comprise the only public organisation in which women play a dominant part. The participation of women in such healing groups has been argued to 'allow the voice of women to be heard in a male-dominated society, and occasionally enable participants to enjoy benefits to which their status would not normally entitle them' (Corin and Bibeau, 1980).

Here, the representation within the illness itself of what we might feel is its aetiology – gender inequality – extends also to the healing group. While there are parallels with psychoanalysis and shamanism, in both of which transcending one's own difficulties confers the ability to help others, a closer analogy is perhaps that of self-help organisations such as Alcoholics Anonymous, or perhaps contemporary women's therapy groups. No social institution need remain restricted to its original rationale, and, just as anti-drug groups such as Synanon and the American Mental Health Movement each transformed themselves from a self-help group into something we may regard as a politico-religious sect, so have the 'hernia societies' of Zaire moved beyond mutual support to adopt a powerful social role, including rights over tax collection (Janzen, 1978). 'Self-help' groups of this type, in the industrialised West or elsewhere, seem to share a similar ideology in which the problem is recognised to be a continuing vulnerability rather than something for which the group can claim to effect a radical cure. Thus we find them associated with medicine's 'chronic disorders', such as alcoholism, vitiligo, epilepsy and cystitis.

Gender politics: men

Saka and sar appear to articulate and resolve, at least temporarily and for the individual, gender oppositions which become manifest as something we might call 'tensions'. Men appear to be less subject to 'psychopathology', either because as the dominant group they have less access to such patterns than do women who are already identified as vulnerable to sickness or possession, or else because they are less 'stressed', having access to everyday mechanisms of power to adjust their difficulties. The distinction may be difficult to draw. As with overdoses, when do 'symptoms' become 'strategies'? Much seems to depend on the local meanings. In certain situations men, of course, become depressed or possessed: situations in which, I would argue, they have lost access to everyday male power. This may occur in situations where young men, in order to marry, are forced into dependence on their fathers-in-law or their kin, as in the New Guinea Highlands (Littlewood and Lipsedge, 1987); or where they take an overdose when unemployed. At times they may be hoist with their own petard of male authority, as are those young men in Morocco who are unable to live up to the ideals of male virility through suffering impotence, physical weakness or deafness (Crapanzano, 1973). Again, the disabling power, the *jinn*, is conceived of as female and as jealous of men: here, she is placated to achieve a cure and is explicitly involved in treatment. The resolution is achieved by her transformation from 'a force disruptive to the social and moral order into a force to preserve that order. So long as her follower obeys . . . his society's moral code, she enables him to live up to the idea of male dominance, superiority and virility' (Crapanzano, 1973).

To seek for 'therapy' or its analogues where we have patterns which are implicitly modelled on physical sicknesses (as in general psychiatry) is plausible. There is a similar situation with 'possession states'. Western psychiatry has long justified itself through the argument that the European 'witches' of the early modern period were really hysterical women whose appropriate treatment was the proper concern of psychiatry (Spanos, 1983), and parallels have been drawn between European treatment of those identified as witches and the procedures of psychiatry (Szasz, 1971). From bewitchment to possession states and thence to multiple personality was a short step, given the whole complex of popular European beliefs in spirit familiars and so on. This is not to mention the ethnocentric titillations provided by dealing with the exotic (as a voyeur) only to reduce it to psychopathology (thus reaffirming our scientific world after all). If we are justified in considering local patterns of understanding in terms of something which can be called a 'spirit' or 'soul' (even if, as I have argued above, these are collective representations akin to the faculties of academic psychology), we must also consider other patterns of dislocation and adjustment which are not locally explained as anything like an 'illness' at all. To search merely for approximate parallels to Western therapies, identifying something akin to them in other societies and then to claim that 'therapy' as we know it is universal, involves what Kleinman and Sung (1979) call a 'category fallacy'. By this means we omit the full range of local meanings, concentrating on a selected core to prove our case in advance.

From rite to illness

If, in the West, we feel uncomfortable with considering overdoses, shoplifting and baby-snatching simply as 'cultural' patterns, seeking to find behind them the 'real' (psychological) determinants, then in any attempt at comparison we need to examine patterns which may be embedded in local understandings quite different from those of 'illness'. Calendrical rituals like communal celebrations at certain times of year, or rites of passage during certain life transitions, are usually excluded from consideration as 'therapy' even though the local exegesis may closely link them.

In Trinidad, the annual carnival is described as a necessary opportunity to release pressure, a healthy catharsis which prevents *grinding* (building up worries and anger inside oneself [Littlewood, 1988]). Trinidadians argue that carnival determines the local personality, one they see as more phlegmatic and adaptive than that of other West Indians. Some anthropologists (e.g. Loudon, 1959) have argued that communal rituals which express existing 'tensions', and resolve them through a constrained manifestation, may in the breakdown of pre-industrial social formations become attenuated into individual patterns which we ourselves might term 'neurotic'. Loudon's example is the periodic rite of *nomkubulwana* among the Zulu in which, at the time of the new crops, women not only celebrated the fertility of the land but also, during a limited period, gave expression to their resentments against men, a pattern which certainly demonstrated local antagonisms between the sexes but 'resolved' them ceremonially for a time at least (Gluckman, 1963). By the middle of this century, the ceremony could no longer be performed. The social structure had been drastically altered as the men now had to leave their homes for up to two years at a time to seek work in the urban areas of Durban and Pietermaritzburg. The women perforce became the household heads in their absence and started to demonstrate a pattern of 'anxiety', *ufufunyana*, characterised by preoccupations with childbirth.

Given the scanty information available to the white anthropologist it is unwise to claim a simple 'translation' of shared ritual into unresolved individual psychopathology. The example does, however, suggest that they may at one level be equivalents, while showing how white colonisation not only induces what we might term 'stress' into the system but pathologises the whole social field so that the very idiom in which the relations between the sexes (and races) is expressed becomes one of psychology. And psychology itself is the ideology of the individual, of loneliness and despair, of anxiety and threatened autonomy. We might argue that 'black' or 'women's' or 'men's' 'consciousness raising' groups or other less overtly therapeutic movements might reverse the process, not just by providing 'therapy' for the individual but by reframing the whole field again (e.g. Teish, 1985; Danforth, 1989).

In the Western Pacific island of Tikopia, aggrieved or offended young women swim or take a canoe out to sea when nobody is around. As an islander comments: 'A woman who is reproved or scolded desires to die, yet desires to live. Her thought is that she will go to swim, but be taken up in a canoe by men who will seek her out to find her. A woman desiring death swims seawards; she acts to go to die. But a woman who desires life swims within the reef' (Firth, 1961). The parallels with drug overdoses in Britain or America are striking. Looking at it from the outside, while completed suicide seems to be some sort of revenge on the whole community, the person who survives a suicide swim attains an enhanced status together with a renegotiation of the original problem. Here, the compulsion on others to act is not one derived from sickness or spirit intrusion but from the threat of physical death. Its idiom is one of personal choice and personality, one, we might argue, of pure psychology. How does the protagonist enhance her status? Through the idea of any solo canoe trip being a dangerous venture. Young Tikopians make risky journeys by themselves in a canoe as a test, an achievement, as what we might perhaps simply call a dangerous 'adventure'. The analogues of 'suicide swims' then are not just those of overdoses but of socially deprived male adolescents 'playing chicken' in front of fast traffic or stealing powerful sports cars to 'joy ride' or race along our motorways.

Whether the above are conventionally regarded as 'pathologies' in themselves is uncertain. While certainly regarded as a legitimate concern for the clinical psychologist, they are not accepted as dangerous 'sports' like motor racing or rock climbing, nor have they attained the medical status of the female syndromes of shoplifting or baby-snatching (Littlewood and Lipsedge, 1987). The extent to which we extend our notions of pathology and thus therapy (or punishment if we subscribe to the 'they need discipline, not therapy' model) is hardly predetermined.

Ihembi and the case of Kamahasanyi

If, as I have argued, we cannot assume the universality of something like therapy just by identifying striking instances in non-Western societies which have characteristics recalling those of psychotherapy, then my examples so far have been limited by a too thin description. Processes and parallels can only be recognised in a more contextualised account. Victor Turner (1964) describes a richly embedded therapeutic encounter, one frequently cited and well worth reading in the original. It concerns the experiences of a young man, Kamahasanyi (let us call him K), a member of the Ndembu who live in what is now Zambia. Turner's account describes a series of events that took place in the 1950s. As with the Somali, the Tikopians, and my other examples, we cannot here pretend to any sort of autonomous society untouched by European colonisation. Nor can the descriptions given by anthropologists offer the 'real' situation, for not only do we (and they) have the problem of the observer being a member of the very institutions responsible for colonising, but anthropologists themselves, anxious to show the rationality of the people they write about, frequently slip into an inappropriate use of Western psychology. Turner actually entitled his paper 'An Ndembu Doctor in Practice' and is candid about his close relationship and admiration for his friend, the healer Ihembi.

The Ndembu, we learn, do not make rigid distinctions between the causes of physical sickness, emotional difficulties, bad luck or other misfortunes. Such misfortune is not accepted as 'fate' but as something whose cause must be elucidated and addressed. A common cause of misfortune is the malevolent attention of a dead person, a power we might gloss as a 'shade', bearing in mind that such shades are not something like a disembodied ghost from a Hollywood film but rather potent symbolic condensations of moral values, memories and personal experiences. Our patient, K, has had a variety of recent misfortunes including bad luck and a variety of physical complaints.

The Ndembu trace descent through the mother's line (although property and power are, as elsewhere, invested in individual men) but wives go to live with their husbands.

Already we can identify a likely difficulty. Young men as they achieve adulthood have to leave their parents' house and go back to their mother's village to obtain their inheritance and status; fathers are often reluctant to leave their carefully accumulated property to those who are not their children (to their sister's children in fact), while some young men are reluctant to leave home for an uncertain future with their mother's brother on whom they must make their claim. There are a variety of strategies such as marrying your father's sister's daughter [work it out] which can help fathers avoid this but they are hardly regarded with approval. K had tried this unsuccessfully and after a quarrel with his father's family, he divorced and finally ended up in his mother's village taking with him some unattached relatives of his father. Tensions exist between this group and the rest of K's mother's village and he seems to be stuck in the middle. If he were a more assertive person he could mediate between the two factions, and he even has some claims through birth on the village headship, but he is (as described by Turner) 'snobbish and unfriendly' while so weak that he permits his current wife to have an affair with someone else. In the background are other disputes: the obvious candidate for the village headship has been forced out of the village and the current acting village head is the father of K's erring wife. After consultation with others, K calls in the healer Ihembi who comes from some distance away and, although he is aware of them, is not involved in the village problems. The villagers themselves wonder as to which shade is responsible for all this. Is it that of K's late father, still angry with his son for quarrelling with his kin? Or that of the last tribal chief affecting the village for disputing the succession of its natural head but taking it out on K? Or is it the whites whose colonial power and ownership of the copper mines have eroded traditional values and caused these tensions?

To simply label these three interpretations respectively as 'guilt about the dead father', 'family conflicts' and the 'experience of political and economic stress' would be inappropriate, although we might note that both the Ndembu and our own understanding deal with similar limitations on personal autonomy and with their internal representations for individuals. After telling Turner privately that he thinks the problems are insoluble and that K should leave the village, Ihembi then changes his mind and decides to have a go at resolving the problems. Perhaps K's wife and her lover are also to blame? In the middle of a dramatic session Ihembi makes general statements to the assembled village about the state of affairs, and goes round the key figures, K's wife, her lover, the closest relative to the 'real' head, other villagers, and K himself, persuading them to make public statements that they bear no one any ill will and then, amidst a crescendo of mounting tension, removes from K the shades both of his father and the dead chief. They represent the ultimate causes. There is a general sense of what we might term 'catharsis' – a collective release of tensions and general reconciliation. Returning to the village some time later Turner finds K much better, communal tensions resolved, and the news that the unwelcome group of K's paternal kin have decided to leave.

The shades here were physically represented in the form of incisor teeth, and it is these which are very publicly removed from K by Ihembi at the right moment. Sleight of hand? Yes. Deception on the part of the healer? Yes and no. The public 'extraction' by traditional healers of harmful substances from sick people is often cited by observers as duplicitous nonsense, very different from the insight achieved in psychotherapy. But what is at issue? The healer certainly has a different level of operation from that of the sick person, and he does not share his own reasoning with that sick person. (We have to take it on trust that he does with Turner.) But is this so different from the evasions of the psychotherapist when faced with direct questioning by the patient about his or her technique? Or the strategic double-binds of structural family therapy? Or the general removal of symptoms which condense down into themselves whole levels of personal and collective meaning?

A famous paper by the French anthropologist Claude Lévi-Strauss looks at the question in the case of a Central American shaman. The shaman, when questioned by the anthropologist, observes that the process of therapeutic change is not physical (the patient, he says, 'believes strongly') but that to make it more effective he represents it to his clientele as something physical; besides, as a successful practitioner, he has to keep his professional knowledge to himself (Lévi-Strauss, 1968a). The limits of what constitutes an acknowledged 'placebo', in other words the 'social' meaning of healing, are uncertain in any context. Doubtless other shamans view it differently. As do psychotherapists.

What is a cure anyway?

Turner's account of healing among the Ndembu places great emphasis on the 'healing' of a whole group through dealing with the illness of an individual in whom the shared problems are most clearly manifest. He is obviously influenced by Ihembi's own explanations to him. At the comparative level, how much can we ignore the changes in others involved in order to concentrate on the designated patient? To an extent this is our Western problem. Kleinman and Sung (1979) argue that traditional healers do best at treating illness, while biomedicine does best with disease, unless it is chronic disease when Western medicine comes under attack for failing to pay attention to continuing distress (illness). Our Cartesian distinction between the (patient's) illness and the (doctor's) disease makes it difficult for the psychotherapist to rest content with 'non-specific' factors of empathy or social context (such as medical power manifested in the high technology hospital, constrained physical contact or white coat and stethoscope): they are merely a 'placebo'. Let us admit that the psychotherapist models himself on the doctor, but in attempting to become 'scientific' and divest himself of these non-specific factors (which embody at one level the context of his privileged authority), he divests himself similarly of what he takes as only the trappings of science to examine the 'real', context-independent, intrapersonal changes.

This is certainly the position of Freud. A more socially contextual approach is that of Freud's one-time rival, Pierre Janet, who in his 1925 treatise *Psychological Healing* traces the development of his own psychological theories of dissociation and 'psychological economy' from European folk healing, through eighteenth-century notions of magnetism to Christian Science, and thence to Charcot, Freud and himself. In part because Janet never attained, outside France, the influence of Freud, and in part because the phenomena with which he was principally interested, dissociation and multiple personality, disappeared as fashionable pathologies, his comparative approach fell into neglect. By contrast, the psychodynamic mechanisms postulated by Freud were enthusiastically taken up in America to explain how traditional healers might effect changes in their patients.

The efficacy of psychoanalysis was said to depend on assumptions shared by patient and therapist, and through which the process of cure was the gaining of 'insight' into his or her motives and symptoms. Insight is described, of course, as being the acquisition of some sort of psychoanalytical perspective, a point made much of by generations of opponents (Gellner, 1985). How then could these supposedly universal mechanisms be employed by the shaman, ignorant as he was of the Freudian *corpus*? The solution has been to contrast the shaman's only partial relief (symptomatic, suggestion, placebo, etc.) with full psychoanalytical insight which precluded any recurrence of the symptoms. The psychoanalysts took up the criticisms of 'suggestion' levelled against them by medical opponents of psychoanalysis (such as Sargant, 1957) to turn them against the traditional healers. Georges Devereux (1970) goes so far as to argue that the traditional healer is himself actually psychotic (in something called his 'ethnic unconscious') and is cured 'without insight' through becoming a healer. Ari Kiev, an American psychiatrist, edited an influential collection of essays published in 1964 entitled *Magic, Faith and Healing*. In his introduction he takes the notion of 'psychotherapy' as unproblematic when employed across cultures, but argues that it is 'primitive psychotherapies' which are universally found. 'Primitive psychotherapy' is his term for psychotherapy as it was before Freud. Its procedures are those of 'suggestion' and 'imitation'. The psychodynamic mechanisms are those disparaged by Freud: projection of personal character-istics onto others (here, the explanation of sorcery), or Fenichel's 'transfer-ence neurosis'.

More modestly, Jerome Frank's *Persuasion and Healing*, published in 1961, tried to select out certain universal features of therapy. In the revised form (1971) they comprise the following: a socially recognised healer who has a superior status to the patient and who is trained in a particular technique; a shared model of explanation; a new perspective offered to the patient; mobilisation of the patient's sense of hope; provision of experiences of success in therapy, and facilitation of 'emotional arousal'. By contrast with the psychoanalytical view, Frank's factors are so general that he questions whether 'psychotherapy' is not just some special case of 'healing' in general. Fuller Torrey (1971) offers a similar schema in which he emphasises the 'cultural congruence' between healer and patient, while Raymond Prince (1976) also argues that healing systems are really systematic elaborations of already existing ways of solving personal problems, such as enacting one's dreams in daily life and other preoccupations. Thomas Scheff (1979) emphasizes parallels with theatre: dramatic re-enactments of personal problems which are resolved 'out there', for principal and audience alike.

A rather literary and much criticised account of shamanic healing is that by Lévi-Strauss (1968b) which describes a woman in obstructed labour among a Central American Indian community. Resolution of the problem involves the shaman in the recitation of a myth about a quest to find the abode of the power which is responsible for the formation of the fetus. The prolonged labour implies the power has exceeded its functions and will not release the child out into the human world. The recitation is lengthy and involves the manufacture and dramatic deployment of small figures representing the protagonists whose symbolic meanings are expressed in appropriate forms, colours, textures and materials. Together, patient and healer participate in a common quest in a shared cultural idiom, linking current physiology (obstructed birth) with its cognitive representation. The healer 'rapidly oscillates between mythical and physiological themes, as if to abolish in the mind of the sick woman the distinction which separates them' (Lévi-Strauss, 1968b: page 193).

Tantalisingly vague as to the actual mind/body interactions (refusing thus to subscribe to our Western Cartesian reasoning but at the cost of what has been taken as mysticism), Lévi-Strauss returns to the original Freudian question of 'hysteria', or, more generally and less pejoratively, to how bodily symptoms occur in relation to popular understanding of them rather than in relation to underlying pathophysiological processes. This is certainly a problem where distress is presented in a somatic form (Chapter 1). Current psychodynamic thinking, however, like general psychiatry, rejects the idea of any standardised relationship between, say, organ and psychological complex: there is no intrinsic association between illness and disease, or at least no causal association from the former to the latter. The emergent meaning of 'the disease' is one derived from popular association and personal cogitation (aided, it is true, by the psychotherapist's emphasis on meaning). Even Kleinman and Sung's (1979) critique of Western medicine is still resolutely Cartesian, leaving non-Western therapies to deal with the biologically 'non-specific' alone. We seem to have a general Western consensus, both medical and psychotherapeutic, that physical symptoms are either a consequence of a disease process mediated through a general notion of 'stress' (whether physiological, emotional or social), or else a shaping of the existing patterns of 'arousal' (such as the psychophysiology of anxiety) through selective attention and positive feedback. Or both. Therapy is seen as reducing stress in the first model and as cutting through feedback in the latter.

This consensus is perhaps one of mechanism rather than of meaning and it does seem to miss the rich symbolic (body + mind + spirit + society) forms of many systems of non-biomedical healing. Is it inevitable for anything we can call therapy? A framework in which we can explore the issues further is that of Dow (1986), perhaps the most useful example of current anthropological thinking. Dow proposes the general term *symbolic healing*. It has, he argues, four general stages, as enumerated below. (I have modified and elaborated his argument somewhat):

(1)   The experiences of healer and healed are already found in a generalised form in a set of 'deeper', shared, culturally meaningful schemata we can call myths, in which symbols couple together personal experience with the social order. Life is experienced through such myths which contain certain accepted (and possible) notions of individual identity, personality and action.

(2)   A suffering individual comes to the healer who defines the presenting problem for the patient in terms of the myth, not just explicitly but through behaviours which recall and make real the myth for the individual. This procedure might be either what we would term physical or non-physical, but it does employ the existing assumptions about the physical (or non-physical) nature of mythic interactions and precipitating experiences, including notions of causality and time.

(3)   The healer transfers the patient's personal emotions, which are still bound up with the problem, onto transactional symbols particularised, as the case demands, from the general myth. This might involve direct

instruction, clarification, confrontation, example, paradox, downplaying other procedures, or through the patient forming an attachment to some figure which encapsulates the myth.
(4)   The healer manipulates these transactional symbols to assist the patient to transact his or her emotions.

If this too seems a little general it is perhaps because we are embedded in our own myths (say, those of bourgeois self-actualisation and autonomy) which are both powerful and yet implicit. To reverse the usual processes by which we measure others' therapies (here, of course, we use 'myths' in the pejorative sense: we have science, they have myths, therefore their therapy is illusory) by our own procedures and to look at our own myths is not to invent some novel approximation to a tribal myth, but to recognise that intersubjective cultural world into which any person is born and in which he or she lives[2]. We can certainly examine empirically how the different bits work: how collective understandings have a certain relationship to social processes; how individuals are socialised into them; how certain themes come to the fore with different types of distress; even whether healing 'works' within its constraining circle of problem and understanding. The way the whole process hangs together, and thus its power, remains however at the level of interpretative rather than empirical study. To say that in general 'therapy works' is a question of the same order as asking whether marriage or religion or democracy 'works'; of making higher order assumptions in which self, others and problem are articulated within an overarching system of meaning which encompasses what it is to be human.

Repression, possession, oppression

The comparative perspective is a necessary one in order to get outside the limits of our own immediate preoccupations and to recognise the context of our own procedures – and their power. It would be unwise, however, to see non-Western systems of healing as being enclosed, always acceptable, unitary processes within a society. As societies change and are in conflict, therapeutic routes themselves change and also may be in conflict; nor are the boundaries of a society or its therapy invariate. Thus, the obvious first option for intercultural work – to continue to provide some accessible form of 'traditional healing' (Reynolds, 1976; Kiev, 1986; Shook, 1985; Laguerre, 1987) – looks dubious. On the Dow model, our deep myths cease to have the power they might once have had. A multicultural society already embodies competing realities, for dominant and sub-dominant alike: pluralist, consumerist, polyphonic.

The second option, a simple move to the dominant Western therapies, is problematic, not only because of the practical and political questions outlined in Chapter 1, but because our collective myth, whatever its representations in advertising, the media and in economic structures, is hardly one whose subjective experience by individuals of different ethnic groups is uniform. The third general schema, that of intercultural therapy as outlined in this volume (see also Ikechukwu's excellent paper (1989)) involves some under-standing of both the first two options – so called 'traditional representations' and 'Western' ones – but by its acknowledgement of context not only allows some synthesis or movement between the two but, more significantly, recognises the pluralistic context in order to develop a dynamic therapy in which the myth is itself one of transformation: in the currently favoured idiom, one of 'growth'. Not then a reassertion of the healing of small-scale pre-industrial societies, for we do not live in one, but a 'Western' therapy. In part, a 'psychological' therapy. And yet one which is fully cognisant of its powers.

Let us take the instance of payment for therapy. Within conventional individual psychotherapy, money not only provides a convenient form of livelihood for the therapist and one which is congenial to his or her assumptive social position as a middle-class professional – the nexus of the activity – but it takes on its own symbolic transformation in the course of the therapeutic encounter, articulating not only the developing relationship between therapist and patient, but intense personal (and sometimes bodily) meanings. We cannot separate out the act of payment in the transaction from its associated meanings. Money, as an abstracted representation of social relations in most encounters between people, carries with it an assumption of individual autonomy, complementary, enhancement of interiority (and of psychologisation) and thus implies a taboo on physical touching and a repression of the biological. For therapists who are united with their patients in a struggle against any form of 'racism', symbolically and instrumentally, 'free' therapy at centres such as Nafsiyat becomes part of shared assumptions about power and about constraints on autonomy which are rather different from those that prevail in Hampstead. As of course does the funding of the Nafsiyat Centre by the local health authority. And these too carry within them particular notions of the self and of change which are not just external constraints, but part of their myth.

The last but related option is that some quite novel schema is devised, one that is experimentally powerful for both therapist and patient, and whose understandings derive from 'the experience of power in a racist society' (Moodley, 1987), where self-hood and actualisation have been represented through a myth which is more congenial to the dominant group and which when represented in the oppressed only offers an identity and goals which are taken as inherently flawed, defined from the outside. Such a therapy of what might be termed resistance, may be said to be inherent in existing forms of intercultural therapy, or it may be elaborated in a new form similar to women's therapy groups (Teish, 1985). The transactional symbols of 'possession' (appropriation of authenticity) might well make more sense than those of 'repression'. Or of 'oppression'. Our brief comparative survey would argue that it is only likely to be developed in its fullest form in contexts where healer and healed share a common schema, in which the individual life of each develops its meaning through its evolving relationship to the other.

Notes

(1) It is, of course, just as arbitrary a construction to select certain biological patterns as the disease (Littlewood, 1991).
(2) The use of the term 'myth', in non-religious and in Western contexts, to connote those shared 'deep' experiential and cognitive worlds which legitimate current action, is argued in Littlewood and Lipsedge (1987). (See also Leach, 1976.)

Part II: Interpretations

Chapter 4

Interprofessional Consultation: Creative Approaches in Therapeutic Work Across Cultures

DEREK STEINBERG

To work psychotherapeutically across cultures is usually perceived as something of a challenge; after all, misunderstandings are common enough, where problematic feelings and behaviour are concerned, even within the same culture. When more than one professional discipline is involved together (psychiatrist and social worker, surgeon and counsellor, psychologist and teacher or even larger combinations) the act of trying to organise, co-ordinate and maintain help can feel like really quite difficult work across conceptual divides. It is at such times that the approaches and methods of interprofessional consultative work between professions can be helpful.

Later on in this chapter, I will describe interprofessional consultation in a little more detail. For the moment, it may be defined as the work done when one person, the *consultant*, helps another, the *consultee*, to use his or her own ideas, perspectives and methods more effectively; the consultant doesn't take over, but starts from where the other worker is, and this requires, above all, imagination.

It constitutes a special way of working, with relevance to working across ethnic cultures *and* conceptual cultures, whether with clients or colleagues. It is distinctive enough, I believe, to justify its own name and identity, but it has also to be admitted that the same term is used for many other things too, often markedly different – for example, in clinical consultation, when a doctor prescribes treatment or gives direct instructions. This is, of course, an important way of working with people's problems, but it is the opposite of consultation as the term is used here. Because of a requirement to clear a space and role for itself, the term 'consultation' has come increasingly to refer particularly to work between professionals (Caplan, 1970; Gallessich, 1982; Steinberg and Yule, 1985). I have proposed elsewhere that consultative work between professional workers be identified as 'interprofessional consultation' (Steinberg, 1989) and suggested that, in addition, it is worth affirming the general notion of a consultative approach for *any* work where people help others to use their own resources rather than applying their own. For example, as will be seen later, much of the worker–client activity described as counselling comes into this category. This is not true of *all* counselling, however (interpretive psychotherapy, for example), hence the room for misunderstanding. In this chapter, various applications of a consultative approach in general, and interprofessional consultation in particular, will be discussed in relation to work in the intercultural therapeutic field.

Consultation described

The consultative approach in general may be defined (as above) in terms of one person, the consultant, helping another, the consultee, with a problem or issue. This is done without imposing the consultant's perspectives and methods, and without any sense of the consultant 'taking over' from the consultee.

This approach requires the consultant to have a proper degree of regard and respect, appropriate to the matter in hand, for the consultee. This last qualification is important and the following two brief vignettes are given by way of example. One is from the field of interprofessional consultation, the other from consultation in a more general sense.

Example 1

A psychologist is asked to take a consultative group for staff of a Children's Crisis Centre. Her task is to help the staff develop good child care and social work practice in a setting where the clientele come from many different cultural backgrounds. Soon after the first two meetings have got under way it becomes clear that the principles the consultative group are developing stand little chance of being put into practice. This is due to the fact that the senior staff responsible for longer term policy-making, planning and training are not involved in the consultation, even though they have given the scheme a genuinely meant go-ahead 'in principle'. A new start has to be made, and new negotiations about the programme and participation in it undertaken with senior staff.

Example 2

A white psychiatrist is referred a teenage girl from an Asian family. She is threatening suicide because of her distress and opposition to a marriage proposed by her parents. The male psychiatrist finds his own feelings very mixed, and his understanding of the facts and nuances of 'arranged marriages' deficient. An exchange of understanding takes place, the psychiatrist contributing his clinical and family work skills, and his acknowledgement of the 'pull' on the girl from two different sets of values. Members of the family in the meantime are able to speak for their own cultural expectations, and from this the psychiatrist learns a great deal. He finds, for example, that there is, in the family, far more understanding of and sympathy with the girl's own wishes and feelings than there seemed to him at first sight. He is able to incorporate this helpfully in the therapeutic work.

In the first instance, the consultant went into the work at the wrong level, since the aim (development in policy and staff skills) wasn't within the power and authority of the consultees. In the second, the psychiatrist held a fine balance between his clinical authority and the need to learn how this family in this culture operated. From what he learned by consulting the family, he was able to respect the family's position, to the young woman's ultimate advantage. In a quite different sort of case, however, there could have emerged evidence of a young person being ill-treated behind a cloud of secrecy and evasion mistakenly attributed to 'tradition', and the option of consulting with the family on an equal and equitable basis would not have been feasible.

Any approach in which A helps B explore a problem means that both learn in the process. The educational component of consultative work is crucial to its principles, its methods, and indeed its raison d'être. Figure 4.1 conveys

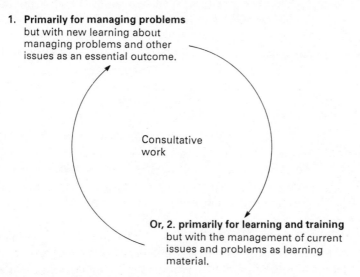

1. **Primarily for managing problems** but with new learning about managing problems and other issues as an essential outcome.

Consultative work

Or, 2. **primarily for learning and training** but with the management of current issues and problems as learning material.

Fig. 4.1   The dual role of consultation.

something of this, in that the consultation may be *primarily* to do with dealing with a problem, but with new learning as an anticipated result too. Alternatively, the consultation may be set up primarily as an educational or training exercise, with day-to-day problems (and ways of tackling them) as the material from which the people involved, consultant and consultees alike, learn. (The first example, given above, might have proceeded along these lines.) Thus the consultative approach can be used in any training exercise where the consultant acts as facilitator to help people with different skills use them collaboratively to explore a theme (examples can be found in: Steinberg, Wilson and Acharyya, 1989; Steinberg, 1991).

We should not perhaps be too surprised that the concept of consultation can challenge the distinctions between professional and client, expert and 'non-expert'.

If we include certain sorts of worker–client relationship (i.e. some forms of counselling) under the general rubric of consultative work then the following are other examples of how consultation may happen in practice:

(1)   A group representing an ethnic minority makes itself available to anyone, professional or general public, who wants to know more about the community and how to relate to its members.

(2)   An individual or group in an area which has recently received a large number of refugees from another country makes itself available both to the community in general and to the health and welfare authorities, and offers help in crises of misunderstanding, problems in the use of services, and in the form of educational workshops. This is sometimes known as a 'culture broker' (Littlewood and Lipsedge, 1989).

(3)   A doctor is trying to help a patient who has a chronic, incurable disease where the patient wants to use a remedy supplied by a traditional healer. The doctor knows nothing about this particular remedy and fears the worst. She consults a health worker from the patient's community to find out the pros and cons and general standing in local terms of what the patient wants to try.

(4)   A hospital receives a number of patients from a small minority community about which its staff find they know little. The staff approach leaders of the community to ask for a consultative seminar in which there can be a joint exploration both of issues that arise in their work and the experience and problems that arise from the user's point of view.

(5)   A psychiatrist finds that her patient has begun to see a religious minister of a little known sect. It isn't clear whether this is helpful or not, and whether it conflicts with her own work or not. She consults the patient about the place this religious group occupies in his life, and when this

doesn't deal with her doubts she consults, with appropriate permission, the patient's relatives and other ministers of religion.

(6) A social worker has been treating the unusual behaviour of a client from another culture with a lot of respect, but begins to have doubts. He consults with a junior colleague who comes from the client's country, and learns that his client is in fact behaving in a most bizarre way. The social worker and his colleague then consult with a psychiatrist in order to consider together how far this odd behaviour is within the normal range, whether it amounts to a clinical 'disorder', and if so what the social worker's future involvement should be.

Consultation defined

I hope that the above examples demonstrate the important (perhaps essential) nature of the consultative approach. It amounts to a process of joint exploration within which individuals, with their own areas of expertise, are also aware of the limits of their knowledge. There is thus an exchange of advice and information, each learning from the other, but the responsibility, position and autonomy of those involved are not compromised. What happens next is another matter; consultation may continue, or (as in Example 1), may have to be abandoned while renegotiation takes place. In the case of the girl with the impending marriage, useful therapeutic involvement can follow; in other circumstances (such as child ill-treatment or neglect) clinical work might have to pause while statutory steps are taken to protect a young person.

Consultation, then, provides a means of enabling those involved in a problem to take action in the light of a broader perspective, with more information and better understanding than they would otherwise have had. In this sense consultation is a mode of operating which can, as it were, be 'slipped into' at will to match the needs of a situation as they arise – as, for example, when a clinician, engaged in therapeutic work, suddenly has to hold back to learn more from the patient. But consultation will often be planned and pre-arranged when, for example, a psychiatrist, psychologist, social worker or member of any other appropriate profession conducts a staff group on a regular basis to help with staff training and development. This may take the form of discussion about a particular issue, or consist of a service to which people can bring questions and problems. A good example of this is the service provided by the Nafsiyat Centre (Chapter 2).

At the risk of over-emphasising the point, what is it that makes a teaching programme or workshop 'consultative', when, for example, an expert in a given field comes along to teach? All consultation requires an *exchange*. I can think of two training workshops which I have taken, for example, and to which I contributed my own experience in training, consultation and psychiatry, but which could not have proceeded satisfactorily had the participants not been able to contribute their own expertise. In one instance this was in art, drama and dramatherapy (Steinberg, 1989) and in the other their personal ideas and beliefs about health, spirituality and the soul (Steinberg, Wilson and Acharyya, 1989). The consultant should not enter this relationship merely to pay lip-service, as it were, to the expertise of the consultees. On the contrary, if the consultant feels in his or her bones that he or she 'knows the score' in advance, and isn't genuinely curious about the consultees' perspectives and methods, then care should be exercised because whatever he or she is doing, it may not be true 'consultation' as described here.

Given such diversity of practice around this basic principle, the following guidelines (taken from Steinberg, 1989) may help to keep the notion of consultation, as defined here, on the rails:

(1)   The consultant works *through the consultee* rather than directly with the problem in hand.
(2)   It is the *consultee's* perceptions, understanding, skills, methods and *wishes* which are primarily used, not those of the consultant, except in so far as the consultee wants them brought in. Much of the work is to do with helping the consultees widen their perspectives, and selecting from or reframing their thinking thus far.
(3)   *The consultee remains responsible for the work being done or discussed*; this pertains whether it is a training programme or work with a client's case.
(4)   By the same token the *consultee* decides what use if any to make of the consultation. There is no obligation on the part of the consultee to put things that emerge into practice. In this sense (and in others) consultation differs markedly from supervision or didactic teaching, with either of which it is sometimes confused. These modes are, of course, important in their own ways, but they nevertheless lack the special qualities and advantages of consultation.
(5)   The *consultant's* obligation is to only take on a task which he or she believes is within the limits of the consultee's status and role; thus, by an act of faith and common sense, the consultant treats the consultee as a fully responsible and competent individual within that role.
(6)   As already shown, *new learning* is as integral to the process of consultation as is dealing with the immediate matter in hand. Here, a training programme or practical, immediate, day-to-day job expectations may be used as the basis for teaching.
(7)   It should be remembered that it takes skill and responsibility to be a

consultee in the essentially peer–peer exercise of consultation.

(8) Finally, consultation should be a *useful, pragmatic exercise* rather than a rarefied performance. Indeed, if these guidelines appear to be getting in the way, then this too should be a question for consultation. For example, there are times when the technical knowledge of the consultant may be usefully invoked as a contribution to what remains an essentially consultative exercise.

The value of consultation

Why go to such lengths to define this type of work? The point about this concern for precise words, terms and principles is that many very different things can go on between professionals and their clients, and between worker and worker, and they all affect the authority and autonomy of those involved differently. Moreover, the consultative approach has a number of advantages not shared by other methods (Table 4.1). Not only does it encourage the independence, autonomy and responsibility of the consultee, but it helps the problem to be handled within already established relationships. For example, in a school situation a difficult pupil continues to be managed by the teacher instead of being referred to the psychologist's or psychiatrist's clinic and thereby becoming to a degree institutionalised. The non-consultative option, when needed, however occasionally, still remains open if the consultation process demonstrates that it would be valuable (Steinberg, 1983; 1986).

In addition, the non-didactic, joint problem-solving style which is integral to the consultative approach means that the consultee is likely to become not only more confident about knowing what he or she can handle, and doing so, but more proficient in dealing with that sort of problem in future. Consultation is therefore educational in a way that prescribed advice or treatment would not be. Finally, and by no means least important, the consultant too learns something about the consultee's perspectives and skills. Consultation as here defined is a joint training exercise as well as a joint enquiry which generates questions that can be followed up by more systematic research. Table 4.1 lists these characteristics as they apply respectively to interprofessional consultation and to a consultative approach taken with a client.

Consultation and autonomy

Preserving and encouraging the autonomy and responsibility of the consultee is no small matter, and it is over this issue that consultation, despite its origin

Table 4.1 Some advantages of the consultative approach.

	In interprofessional consultation:	In work with clients:
1	The client, pupil or patient of the consultee stays with the consultee instead of being referred to more specialised care; help is closer to the community, and more modest in scale.	The individual's own strengths and skills, e.g. in managing his or her own life or family are encouraged and enhanced. Help is closer to community, and more modest in scale.
2	If more specialised help is really needed, the reasons are made clear, the goals evident, and agreement negotiated.	As opposite.
3	The professional skills and development of the consultee are enhanced; from a wider perspective, professional training is enhanced and the use of specialist services improved.	The personal strengths and knowledge of the client are enhanced; from a wider perspective, public education is enhanced and self-help encouraged.
4	The consultant learns from the consultee as well as *vice versa*.	As opposite.
5	There is encouragement of more appropriate and economical use of services, for all the reasons given above.	As opposite.
6	To work this way is as much a process of joint enquiry as a way of providing help; it constitutes the beginnings of research by formulating questions which aren't often asked.	As opposite.

and basis in interprofessional work, has important implications for work between professionals and their clientele.

To begin with the traditional clinical model of care, the task here is to establish what is 'wrong' with the patient according to the perspective and expertise of the doctor. I would argue that this approach, namely 'A' recognising what is wrong with 'B' according to the conceptual models within which she was trained, is much more central to the essence of the much maligned 'medical model' than are any notions of physical causality and treatment (Steinberg, 1981; Tyler and Steinberg, 1987). It is true that some psychologists, social workers, and psychotherapists can be dismissive of what they call the 'medical model', yet quite often they have in fact adopted it themselves, both in attributing something 'wrong' with the client according to their understanding of behavioural science, psychodynamic theory, or social systems, and in pursuing a course of action designed and prescribed to correct it (Chapter 3).

The consultative model is altogether different, and indeed quite difficult for professional workers to manage since its requirements are for power sharing, ideas sharing, and furthermore exchange of ideas with the consultee. It is not surprising that Caplan, a pioneer of consultation, but himself trained in psychoanalysis, has pointed out the problems people with a background in dynamic psychotherapy encounter when undertaking consultation because of their preoccupations with motivation rather than behaviour, with 'why?' instead of 'what?' (Caplan, 1970). To quote from my own account of consultative approaches in relation to medical practice (Steinberg, 1989), when the doctor (or any other therapist) takes a consultative approach, the therapist does not abdicate from his or her special responsibility and skills, but instead acknowledges the following three important areas of authority and responsibility:

- *the clinician as expert and authority* in their own speciality, personal views and ethical perspectives;
- *the patient as an expert and authority* on him- or herself, with their own ethical and personal preferences;
- *the responsibility of the doctor to teach and to learn* – to help widen the patient's understanding of health, disorder and treatment as the doctor sees it, and in doing so to learn more about the patient and the patient's understanding of these matters and what the patient wants as well as what the patient is supposed to 'need'.

Rather than blurring the roles of the professional and the patient, the consultative approach in fact clarifies and affirms the position of both. Further, the role of the doctor or other therapist, far from being diminished, is, I believe, enhanced, becoming established through a mutual consultation that rests on a firmer foundation than authority by tradition, by accident, or because of a diploma on the wall.

There are two catches, or potential catches, in all of this. First, as Rack (1982) has pointed out, people from some cultural backgrounds may not have confidence in such a non-directive approach, but expect something more authoritative and solid from the therapist in the way of comment, instruction or prescription. Indeed, many patients may be unaware of such professional approaches to health and illness. There is no obligation, however, on the therapist, as consultant, to remain obstinately non-directive if the patient obviously requires something more directive. After all, he or she would be no more idealistic about simply going along with a patient's own notions however inappropriate they might be. The consultative approach is above all interactive, conversational and concerned with what is practical and possible. It is up to the consultant to offer explanation and to proceed with consultation, while it is up to the consultee what use to make of it. So, consultation should be realistic, and if consultant or consultee find it straying into intuition, allusion, collusion, confusion, or some other potential area of mystery, one or other should take the responsibility of blowing the whistle and reviewing aims, objectives and, in general, what is going on.

If the central task of consultation is to help identify and mobilise the consultee's resources, then the consultant will find the work focusing on three broad areas:

(a)   the consultee's personality attributes and strengths;
(b)   the strength, support and help he or she gets, or reasonably expects, from family, friends and (in the case of interprofessional consultation) from colleagues;
(c)   the consultee's work with their client if work with a client is the issue.

The consultant has a difficult task since he or she must work with these areas, with the consultee's autonomy and responsibility firmly centre-stage. The consultative work should not slip into psychotherapy, and nor should the consultant start advising the consultee on how his or her work situation should be changed. Such things can easily happen, for example, when a consultee's feelings appear problematic, or when there is an obvious management problem at work (commonly, lack of adequate supervision, role clarity, and support). Similarly, when work with a client is the focus, the consultant should help maintain the consultee's perspective, and not begin to attempt history taking or clinical work by proxy. All these issues are important, and often emerge in consultative work (Steinberg and Hughes, 1987); the task of consultation should remain one of helping the consultee decide what is needed rather than for the consultant to see each issue through.

Any constraint added to the above depends on the integrity of the consultee as well as the consultant. Once the consultee is clear about what is causing the problem it is up to them to decide on the appropriate action. This could be, for example, to try to change feelings or attitudes either alone or with outside help, to learn more (perhaps seeking further training), or to try to change an aspect of life at home or at work. The consultant's role is to help the consultee see this, but not see it through. Clarification alone is sufficient achievement. If the consultee decides, for example, that he or she needs personal counselling, detailed education about AIDS, or to go on a management course, that is fine, and it isn't up to the consultant to provide it.

It is this key purpose – namely, working primarily with the perspectives, autonomy and responsibility of the consultee – that distinguishes consultation from other types of work, and it is of particular value where one person works with another whose perspectives, values and methods are different from his own.

Consultation and therapy

The case for the special characteristic and value of the consultative approach can, of course, founder when it comes to the current usage of terms. There is, for example, a great deal of overlap and confusion about terms such as counselling and psychotherapy. Some people regard counselling as essentially a non-directive way of helping other people reach their own decisions (Newsome *et al.*, 1975), while Pedder and Brown (1979), giving a very similar definition, nevertheless regard it as among what might be termed the 'outer levels' of psychotherapy. The carefully established and defined non-directive psychotherapy developed by Carl Rogers (1951; 1961) appears to be variously regarded by its exponents as psychotherapy *or* counselling – as if these were interchangeable terms. I referred earlier in this chapter to psychotherapists as using a 'medical model' approach based on their tendency to perceive problems in their clients according to their own highly specialised, elaborate, and even esoteric concepts, rather than according to those of the client. This type of work has, I believe, its own values, but it is quite different in approach from consultation, and from the client-centred psychotherapy originally described by Rogers. It is not so much that one approach is 'better' than the other, it is simply that they represent quite different tools for different sorts of jobs.

All such semantic and practical problems have to be lived with until there are precise enough techniques to establish their identities and operational methods more clearly. One obligation for the psychotherapist or counsellor who is sympathetic to the consultative approach is to at least know what he or she is doing at any given time, so that, even within psychotherapy itself, it is possible to switch to the consultative mode, as in Example 1, and back again.

Despite the obvious room for confusion, I hope it is clear that there is a case for a consultative approach in which the expertise and not merely the wishes of the other person is assumed and that this has a place in worker–client relationships as well as between professional workers themselves. The key test for the person aspiring to the consultative approach is quite a tough one for professionals who are highly trained and practised in specialised techniques: are you *genuinely* curious about the other person's perspective, beliefs, methods and cultural background (whether the latter refers to another country or another school of thought), and do you *genuinely* want to learn? If in all honesty you are and do not, then you will simply be engaged in that continuing tussle that is universal among those working in the social and psychotherapeutic arts (Steinberg, 1981). If you are and do, and really want to learn what it is like to enter the realm of the consultee, you may be attempting consultation.

In psychotherapy, empathy is crucial but usually employed to help the therapist's understanding: i.e. diagnostically. In consultation, the object of empathy can be to facilitate the process (Rogers, 1961).

Consultation and other types of interprofessional work

Here too there is room for misunderstanding since many people who engage in intercultural work will be working across disciplines in a variety of ways. It is worth reiterating that terms such as consultation, collaboration, liaison work and so on are often used interchangeably or without generally accepted definition (compare, for example, Caplan, 1970; Steinberg and Yule, 1985; Mrazel, 1985; Gelder *et al.*, 1985).

In order to help clarify these issues, I would like to offer the following definitions:

Consultation. The work undertaken when one person, the consultant, helps another, the consultee, by encouraging an approach to solving problems in which the consultee clarifies issues, problems and possible ways forward using their own wishes, perspectives and methods, rather than those of the consultant.

Interprofessional consultation. The work undertaken when one professional worker, acting as consultant, helps another, the consultee, along the same lines as above, and without taking over responsibility for the issue or case which the consultee has raised.

Collaborative work. Collaboration means working together, and need have no more precise meaning. Consultation, including interprofessional consultation, is one form of collaboration. A psychiatrist and a social worker, a psychologist and a paediatrician, or a surgeon and an anaesthetist, may collaborate over someone's care without the work being consultative.

Liaison work. Collaboration between different workers, teams or agencies whose work aims are ordinarily different. Thus the Nafsiyat Centre (see Chapter 2) may liaise with, say, a hospital or an embassy, and out of this liaison systematic collaboration or consultation may develop.

Therapy. Therapy means healing or treatment of a disorder or problem, mending or correcting something which has become damaged or gone adrift. It implies one person's expert skills, and therefore differs from consultation. Nevertheless, a therapist can deliberately foster self-help (self-therapy) through a consultative approach towards the client. In the field of psychotherapy there is the established tradition of 'training therapy'. My own view is that psychological training for personal and professional development is worth distinguishing from psychological therapy for personal difficulties.

Counselling. The term 'counselling' is currently used as a general term for any mixture of information-giving, support and (sometimes) consultation. Brown and Pedder (1979) describe it in terms of an 'outer level' of psychotherapy, involving unburdening, ventilation, and support, 'withholding direct advice' and 'leaving decisions to the client'. I believe the term is most appropriately used when the counsellor has new information to impart, whatever other support or consultation is provided, as is the case in legal, civil rights or health counselling.

Supervision. It is worth distinguishing supervision from consultation whereever the latter is discussed, because they are quite often confused in practice. In supervision, the supervisor is expected to have greater expertise in the matter being discussed, and the supervised person correspondingly lesser expertise; the supervisor takes or delegates a varying degree of the immediate responsibility. This is quite distinct from consultation, but the unwary consultant may be surprised to find how often in practice the difference is not appreciated (Steinberg, 1989).

Teaching and training. I will not embark on a definition of 'teaching' here, but merely point out that an important teaching method comes very close to the consultative approach: that of encouraging the student to ask questions, define problems clearly, and find the answers for him- or herself. Consultation is also complementary to quite different and no less valuable forms of teaching, namely, the giving of direct instructions, the demonstration of how to do things, and so on. As was discussed previously, consultation and training (whether professional development or public education) go hand in hand. Not for the first time, it is relevant to point out that the word doctor originally meant 'teacher'. One could ask whether it is a coincidence that therapists have two main lines of ancestry: priests on the one hand; teachers on the other. Throughout this chapter I have tried to emphasize that if we workers are really to know what we are doing in this ambiguous field, and if we are to have a genuine regard for the other person's life and work, then we should know which side of this inheritance we are making use of.

Conclusions

In this chapter I have spent a lot of time on words and their meanings, and indeed on professional rituals and their meanings. I think this is appropriate in the field of intercultural work, particularly since I am struck again and again by the problems inherent in work across different disciplines even before one considers the wider questions of work across cultures (Steinberg, 1986). After all, the cultures of the surgeon, the psychotherapist, the social scientist and the teacher are all very different, and it is as well to recognise this if we ourselves are to teach and learn among each other as well as with our clientele. For the moment, it is clear to me that among the general specialities in what are termed 'helping and caring' professions, the idea that we speak the same language is an illusion.

I would like to end on an anecdote: it is taken from an experiential workshop for general hospital staff in an English-speaking country with a substantially cosmopolitan population. The hospital had people from many different cultures among its patients and staff, and the latter included a number of interpreters. Interpreting as a discipline in a hospital was new to me. The interpreters seemed a little surprised to have been invited along to be with the clinical professionals at all, and described their work with modesty. As the nature of what they did emerged, its dramatic nature and therapeutic implications came as something of a revelation to the others present, and, to a considerable extent it seemed, to themselves as well. Repeatedly, they stood literally between the physician or surgeon on the one hand and the patient and family on the other, conveying for the first time news about a child, an operation, or a prognosis that was sometimes very bad news indeed. They would convey back the responses and questions of the family as best they could, bearing in mind that they often could only partly comprehend and convey the subtleties of the medical information given, and finding themselves sharing much of the shock and pain of the situation.

I mention the above only as an example, and as a new discovery for me, of people in a very small speciality in a hospital, working with courage, humanity and a degree of bafflement, to bridge one of the many cultural, technical and linguistic gaps in our field. This episode emerged, unexpectedly and with impact, during the course of a 'consultative' workshop. We were all surprised at what we found, the interpreters no less than everyone else. In many of the approaches with which such consultation may be compared, we often know more or less what is coming along. But consultation, if genuine, is full of surprises – and so it should be!

Chapter 5

The Doctor's Dilemma:
The Practice of Cultural Psychiatry
in Multicultural Britain

SOURANGSHU ACHARYYA

'When I use a word,' Humpty Dumpty said, in rather a scornful tone, 'it means just what I choose it to mean – neither more nor less.'
'The question is,' said Alice, 'whether you can make words mean so many different things.'
'The question is,' said Humpty Dumpty, 'which is to be master – that's all.'
Lewis Carroll, *Through the Looking Glass* and *What Alice Found There*.

Ethnicity and culture

The United Kingdom has been a 'multi-ethnic society' for some time. Whether it has also been a 'multi-cultural society' for an equal length of time is perhaps open to question. A basic problem lies, perhaps, in the definition of these two terms: over recent years they appear to have become synonymous for psychiatry as well as for many other disciplines. It is I think important to attempt to distinguish them at the outset.

The word *ethnicity* still refers us back to the putative racial origins of people, to their distinctive physical appearance as it is perceived by themselves and others. The word *culture* on the other hand refers to milieu, the process of living and the system of values and practices shared by particular groups of people. Ethnicity, therefore (except in the case of children born of marriage between groups), remains a relatively static concept for the individual. Culture, by distinction, is dynamic. It is ever-changing and includes a whole gamut of experiences and learning and includes all the distinctive practices of daily living, customs and attitudes. Culture encompasses all of everyday life, from the mundane, such as the type of food eaten, even mealtimes, and clothes, to religious practices and important attitudes to others in terms of age, sex, and social roles. Along with these, it includes the extent to which one can adapt to social changes.

In the UK, numerous cultures have been contributing to 'British society' over a very long period. If one looks closely at the history of the UK, it can be realised that the Norman Conquest (to take an example) created a new culture – one that initially 'co-existed' with (and dominated) the native Saxon culture. Subsequently there occurred a dynamic fusion of the 'new' and the 'old': a single pluralistic culture slowly evolved, added to and enriched by other migrant groups (see below), and it is still evolving. Since the 1950s, a large new cultural dimension has been added – the migration of non-European peoples from the New Commonwealth countries. In the case of the Norman influx, ethnic/racial differences may not have been so obvious, at least at first glance. By contrast, in meeting someone from the New Commonwealth, that person's racial identity (or at least a broad racial identity as 'black') is immediately obvious to the native Briton. Thus the term 'ethnic minority' has come to be used rather than that of 'cultural minority'. The use of the term ethnic minority therefore signals more than a difference of lifestyle. It implies an inability (possibly a refusal) to accept (whether by omission or commission) that people from the New Commonwealth are 'cultural' minorities as are Jewish migrants from Eastern Europe, those who are Catholics as opposed to Anglicans, or Southern Europeans who for generations have migrated into this country. From the psychiatrist's point of view this new group, this 'ethnic minority', are also seen to have brought along with them a particular set of mental health problems, tied up with their ethnicity or race, rather than arising from their cultural background or from the process of adaptation and confrontation within the new cultural milieu.

Doctors and 'transcultural psychiatry'

During the process of training doctors in the UK, medical students, in their short course on psychiatry, are sometimes taught some 'transcultural psychiatry'. This subject broadly deals with psychiatric syndromes arising from various parts of the world and essentially involves fragmentary, and in many cases anecdotal, studies of those peoples whose societies have over the past 200 years been colonised by Europeans. The students are offered a glimpse of such exotic culture-bound syndromes as *windigo* which is defined as a particular kind of 'psychosis' among native North Americans in which the affected person apparently resorts to cannibalism.

On closer examination, it is sometimes found that such accounts are purely anecdotal, or may even be fictitious (Littlewood, 1990). Indeed, there is no evidence to suggest that windigo, for example, ever existed. Frequently cited patterns include episodes of *koro* among Chinese and Indo–Chinese people, in which a male develops the unshakeable belief that his penis is being retracted within his body. Again, taking this as a unitary entity, and by so doing highlighting such an exotic departure from 'European' mental illness, makes exciting reading – but whether or not this makes it a discrete culture-bound syndrome remains questionable. (Purely anecdotally, the last person I myself found to present to doctors with such a belief was a sixteen year-old North London schoolboy, whose family, for as far back as the family-tree could be traced, appear to have been English!)

In the West, psychiatrists have tended, covertly or overtly, to play the 'colonialist game' that their own elected politicians have developed. This process has consisted of devising systems of classification of psychiatric disorders which are essentially home-based. If such categories do not embrace migrant peoples (who do not readily fit in the classification system), these people tend to be segregated into something else. Thus they are seen as suffering from an 'exotic' condition – 'West Indian Psychosis', or 'the Begum Syndrome', for example. This problem, I would suggest, has been amplified by the trend in the former colonies to perceive as the root of the power of their erstwhile colonial masters a new religion called 'science and technology'. This has led these nations to send their brightest young people to the West to be trained in this new craft. Psychiatry has been no exception.

The most distinguished of Third World psychiatrists, the doyens of their profession, are mainly (if not wholly) trained by Western psychiatrists in the prestigious teaching centres of the West. The psychiatric elite of the New Commonwealth has been trained by British psychiatrists in Britain. Therefore, these people on their subsequent return to their own cultures, perceive mental illness along the 'British model', and find difficulty in evolving new ways or methods of examining psychiatric disorders within their own cultures (Chakraborty, 1990).

Hughes (1985) suggests that 'both the labels "atypical psychoses" and "exotic syndrome" imply deviance from some "standard" diagnostic base'. If something is 'atypical' it obviously falls outside the range of what is 'typical'. Similarly, 'exotic' means 'foreign', 'different', or 'deviant' from something that is not exotic, that is something that is familiar and well known. So to use these two categorical labels is to imply that we are dealing with psychiatric (or imputed psychiatric) syndromes that fall outside the scope of known and described (and thus legitimate) phenomena.

The doctor's dilemma

What constitutes the 'scope of known and described phenomena'? The frame of reference might be that embodied in the most recent edition of the

International Classification of Diseases (currently the 9th edn), the latest edition of the Diagnostic and Statistical Manual of Disorders of the American Psychiatric Association (currently DSM-IIIR), or any of the contemporary versions of numerous other formal medical diagnostic systems (Spitzer *et al.*, 1983). Herein lies a problem for the doctor diagnosing and treating mental illness in people from cultural minorities, the problem of the title of this chapter: 'The doctor's dilemma'. One is dealing with a person who comes from a different culture, with an attitude to well-being or illness that is perhaps quite different from that of the examining psychiatrist. In addition, the patient might speak a language other than English as a first language. Even if English is the mother tongue, the language used may be semantically and syntactically different from that of the examining psychiatrist. There-fore, the dilemma which arises for our examining doctor is whether this distress, as presented by the patient, is (a) one of the familiar entities according to standard Western classification systems, or (b) if not, then what is it (Littlewood, 1992b). The doctor's dilemma is in deciding where, in a broad group of symptomatological classification it can be included, or indeed (c) whether this condition truly constitutes a 'psychiatric illness' at all.

Shepherd and Wilkinson (1988), when discussing primary health care and psychiatric epidemiology, make an important point: that if our classificatory schemes have been unsatisfactory, then this may have been in some measure due to the system being developed from the studies of patients admitted into hospital and therefore suffering from the most serious illnesses. They particularly single out affective (mood) illnesses, particularly depression and manic–depression. The current systems of classifications include a wide range of affective disorders but fail to include others. This is certainly true of one of the standard classification systems, the International Classification of Diseases, which contains (in its 9th edn) no fewer than 19 specialised categories of depression but allocates many of them simply to a rag-bag of categories it labels 'other'.

What is seen by the individual (or by the individual's family or community) as complex personal distress has, of course, to be slotted into a neat diagnostic box by the doctor, a personage seen by them as the professional expert who can alleviate this distress. Both sides, the patient and the doctor alike, bring their own preconceptions about the other to the encounter. The patient walks through the door of the surgery or consulting room with assumptions about the doctor's work: these may, of course, in some respect be similar to what the doctor believes his or her role to be. But it may also include a range of other qualities or qualifications which the doctor may feel (justifiably or unjustifiably) is hardly their role, perhaps detailed advice on social and financial matters, for example. Similarly, the doctor may have preconceptions of what constitutes the 'patient-ness' of a person. And it may be difficult to redefine this 'patient-ness' in terms of how the patient – this particular patient – presents themselves.

One of the problems for a patient from a minority cultural group may be that what the patient presents as a problem, and the way it is presented, does not fit easily into the standard European text-book classification that the doctor has so meticulously absorbed, categories which are themselves taken to be culture-free. It has been suggested by Littlewood (1990; Littlewood and Lipsedge 1989), that while people from 'other cultures' are very often slotted into the existing categories of mental disorders developed in the West, the reverse does not happen. The categories therefore remain sacrosanct; the patient either has to be shoe-horned in, or left in some marginal 'exotic' or 'culture-bound' category.

In the UK there have been some recent studies which show marked differences in psychiatric morbidity and treatment between the cultural majority and cultural minorities (see Chapter 1, this volume). One study points out that there is a marked increase in the incidence of diagnosed schizophrenia amongst British-born people of West Indian descent compared with the native white population in Britain (Harrison *et al.*, 1988). McGovern and Cope (1987) found higher rates of compulsory psychiatric admissions of people under the Mental Health Act for immigrants from the West Indies, although British-born West Indians were also over-represented compared with the native white population and South Asians.

Can the high rate of detained West Indian patients be explained simply by an increase in the incidence of schizophrenia? It would be comforting to put these findings together in a neat little box and conclude that a genetic predisposition amongst this ethnic group accounts both for the high rate of schizophrenia and the consequent detention. This hypothesis does not stand up to close scrutiny. Littlewood and Lipsedge (1989) found that excessive detention of West Indians under the Mental Health Act was independent of diagnoses. Ineichen and his colleagues (1984) suggested that no significant differences in voluntary admissions of West Indians are found compared with the white population. When one looks at how the population was diagnosed in McGovern and Cope's paper (1987), there is little detailed description of the process of how the diagnosis was reached except to say that they followed the 'final case note diagnoses' ('schizophrenia, paranoid psychoses, affective disorder, neurosis and personality disorder, drug or alcohol abuse, organic psychoses, drug-induced psychosis, other'). Furthermore, among this population, eight West Indian patients were given a diagnosis of drug-induced psychosis. The drug implicated was cannabis. This diagnosis was not given to any patient from the other ethnic groups although Harrison and his colleagues used diagnoses from the standard international classification systems.

If one looks at the World Health Organisation's International Pilot Study of Schizophrenia (Sartorius *et al.*, 1977) the pattern of schizophrenia across the world – in various centres in Europe, North America, Asia and Africa – is extremely similar. However, when it comes to the outcome of 'schizophrenic illness' across the world, there are differences. In the Third World countries, the prognosis appears to be markedly better than in the West. The authors comment that this is due, perhaps, to social reasons. Now, in medicine, 'a disease entity' is marked not only by common aetiology (causes), pathogenesis (disease process), symptoms but also by prognosis. This is particularly so for schizophrenia. However, in the case of schizophrenia, although the International Pilot Study finds markedly different prognoses in different societies, it still adheres to the diagnosis of 'schizophrenia' for these conditions in the Third World societies rather than to question the soundness of the diagnosis of schizophrenia (Kleinman, 1987).

There is some evidence to suggest that when mental illnesses are taken out of the hospital-derived context (which is where the classificatory systems were conceived), identification of symptoms in the case of people from cultural minorities does not follow the same trend as has been found by Harrison and his colleagues (1975), or McGovern and Cope (Chakraborty, 1990). Recent community-based studies, carried out at the Nafsiyat Intercultural Therapy Centre (Chapter 6) found that, (a) the largest single group of the patient population consisted of people who referred themselves to the Centre rather than those referred through the usual statutory services such as general practitioners or hospital psychiatric emergency clinics, and (b) that contrary to the findings of other community 'walk-in' mental health centres (Bouras 1982; 1983; Lim 1983; Hutton 1985), the majority of patients were suffering from severe affective disorders which, according to the usual classification systems, would warrant categorisation as 'affective (depressive) disorder' (Chapter 10). About 19% of their population were suffering from what would be described as psychoses (Acharyya *et al.*, 1989; Moorhouse *et al.*, 1989), but a high proportion of these people had a series of adverse life events during their lives such as separation from parents (especially the mother) at an early age, sexual and physical abuse, and emotional conflicts within their own families (Chapter 8).

It has been suggested both by McGovern and Cope (1987) and by Littlewood and Lipsedge (1989) that what causes minority patients to be labelled as suffering from schizophrenia might have something to do with the manner in which they present their distress. Behaviour which perhaps appears to the observer as 'bizarre', involving verbal or non-verbal patterns which are interpreted as aggressive, implies to an observer from another culture that not only is this behaviour abnormal, but it also indicates schizophrenia. Particularly in the West, since the notion was first introduced by Kraepelin and Bleuler, 'schizophrenia' has signified to lay people, as well as the medical profession, mental disorder of a very profound degree.

We might wonder whether the observer, even the trained observer, observing behaviour in another person from a different culture which is 'bizarre', perhaps talking with them through an interpreter, could be tempted into diagnosing 'schizophrenia' more readily than, say, affective (emotional) disorder. Since the international systems of classification are so vague about defining and classifying affective disorder, but, on the other hand, so certain when describing and defining schizophrenia, it is perhaps small wonder, that when in trouble (i.e. when the patient is not understandable), the doctor may turn more readily to the box marked 'schizophrenia' into which to fit the patient.

If this is so, how does one escape this stereotyping which I have suggested is the neo-colonial practice of psychiatry? It might prove to be an appropriate starting point to view the problem no longer as one of 'transcultural psychiatry' but simply as one of 'cultural psychiatry' in that psychological distress in all societies and groups is equally cultural, equally biological. Perhaps one could also concentrate more on how to help alleviate the distress rather than on wondering what exactly 'it' is.

On the question of epidemiology, we need to take a bird's-eye view of psychiatry. Instead of carrying out inexhaustible exercises in which we reduce entities down so that we can enclose them in boxes of ever-diminishing sizes, we need to take a more open-ended view of concepts, to allow more elbow room for concepts to develop rather than smaller boxes for them to shrink into. The newer multiaxial classification, in which diagnosis is considered together with the person's personality, physical health and preceding life stresses, has been widely welcomed by psychiatrists and other mental health professionals all over the world (Littlewood, 1992b).

Multiaxial classifications still lack, however, the acceptance of cultural variation within societies as well as across societies. Our world has become much more multicultural than it ever has been, due to faster communication and transport, an international economic system, and the consequent migration of peoples. Perhaps it is important for us, when attempting to understand 'the patient', to concentrate harder on actually listening to what the patient is saying in their own terms – whether verbally or non verbally – and to take special note of the particular cultural dimensions that make up personhood. The preconceptions about each other that both doctor and patient bring to their consultation will have to be examined and a dialogue can then take place which may go towards alleviating the patient's distress. In mutually divesting the other of their preconceptions, the doctor has a special role in allowing the patient to feel that they have the power and the right to present their own view of what is wrong. Although the doctors may or may not agree with the patient's constructs, they need to accept such constructs as legitimate, worthy of being given a place in the clinical dialogue. It is the doctor who needs to initiate such a sense of dialogue rather than of confrontation with the patient.

A major difficulty in continuing any such dialogue may be what I would describe as the 'cultural divergence' between the professional and the patient. Every human being, when suffering distress, initially attempts to define the nature of this distress and what may have caused it, and to make sense of it. Once the person has reached a decision (whether this is medically 'correct' or 'incorrect' is immaterial), then the person actively chooses to find appropriate means to alleviate the distress. If, for example, a person with abdominal pain attempts to define the cause of the distress and concludes that because it comes in spasms, in periodic bursts, it is caused by the attacks of a malevolent spirit, then he or she might choose a priest or an exorcist as the most appropriate agent to alleviate this distress. On the other hand, the medical professional may conclude that this is a colic, caused by an inflammation of the gut, and simply prescribe an anti-inflammatory drug. On biomedical criteria the professional may be 'right' and the patient may be 'wrong', but, unless the professional can initiate a dialogue, no joint collaboration in attempting to alleviate the distress can take place. The patient may instead go off to find an exorcist while, in terms of the therapeutic programme, the professional complains about the 'non-compliance' of the patient.

In order to develop my point, a simple diagram may be useful (Fig. 5.1). The central column represents the process by which help is sought for distress. The left hand column represents the professional who, using their cultural constructs (such as medical or social work training), determines what the appropriate means of dealing with the distress might be. On the right we have the person who is experiencing the distress: they too use a cultural construct (which would include their own value systems and understanding of illness as well as the degree of suffering) in order to come to some conclusion about both the nature and the cause of the distress, and who and what would be the appropriate means of alleviating it in order to be well again.

Figure 5.1 demonstrates what in this context I understand as 'culture', a system of understanding which provides both the definition of distress and the appropriate means of resolving it. The left column, under the heading 'professional', demonstrates the way that the professional thinks about such distress; here, for the sake of simplicity, I have chosen the professional to be a doctor. The doctor's own term for the immediate distress is 'the symptom' that 'the patient' (i.e. 'the person') has presented to the doctor. From the cluster of symptoms, the doctor diagnoses 'a disease', for which they would prescribe 'treatment', in order to seek a 'cure of the disease'. The individual on

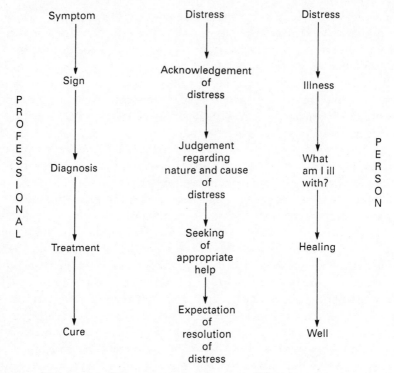

Fig. 5.1   Diagram to illustrate patient-doctor collaboration.

the other hand does not present symptoms but suffers from 'distress' from which the person understands 'I am ill'. The person looks for 'healing' to make the person 'well' again. In this process, the person too is pulled by a particular cultural bias. Instead of being pulled further and further away from the other through cultural constructs, an attempt must be made to build a bridge across the two separate positions, to hold a dialogue in which an attempt at successful alleviation of the distress can begin to take place.

With the power that is invested generally by society (which ultimately includes all of us as potential 'patients') in the professional, and that invested by the specific professional training, it is only too comfortable for the professional to remain in the position of power and to retain a position of supremacy, of prescribing the forms of understanding and treatment to the patient. As this reprehensible if not iniquitous distribution of power remains, then so does the 'doctor's dilemma'.

Chapter 6

Quantitative Research in Intercultural Therapy: Some Methodological Considerations

SHARON MOORHOUSE

In this chapter I will review some of the questions raised by the existing research literature on intercultural therapy which are relevant in any attempt to assess its efficacy.

Three fundamental issues come to the fore. One is the problem of how any psychotherapy can be evaluated. Secondly, how sensitive is the theory and practice of psychotherapy to the needs and experiences of patients from cultures that are different to those of Western Europe? Lastly, how does the concept of 'free' psychotherapy fit into traditional psychotherapy practice, with particular reference to people who may be too ill to work, or who are unable to find work? I shall attempt to illustrate these themes with some of the research findings from a study funded by the Department of Health and carried out at the Nafsiyat Intercultural Therapy Centre (Moorhouse *et al*, 1989).

Quantitative research in this area is complex, and it is important to recognise at the outset the limitations of the existing terminology and to define those terms which we are going to use.

Terminology

There are fundamental differences in how professionals style their particular area of expertise. The words *cross-cultural* or *transcultural* (the latter a term especially used by psychiatrists in the UK) can variously imply work with migrants, with the British-born children of those migrants, or with those whose parents are of different cultures from each other. This confusion has implications for any attempts to carry out research in these areas since there is at present a lack of distinction between these different groups – groups who might be expected to present with rather different problems, experiences and assets.

The term *transcultural* also refers to diagnostic schemata considered across cultures, particularly the so-called 'culture bound syndrome' such as the psychiatrists' favourites *koro* and *amok* (Chapter 5), and also to the ability (or otherwise) of a clinician from one culture to make a diagnosis for a patient from another culture (Westermeyer, 1985; Littlewood, 1990). Implicit here is the assumption that the professional him- or herself does not come from a minority background.

A major advantage in using the term *intercultural therapy* is that it acknowledges the fact that professionals themselves come increasingly from minority backgrounds. Thus it is not only white professionals who need to be proficient in working with people from backgrounds different to their own.

We need also to clarify what we mean by 'race', 'culture' and 'ethnic minority'. The existing literature sometimes confuses these three terms, or uses them interchangeably (see Fernando, 1991 for a further discussion of this).

Race is a term that has largely been discredited in biological science, but was particularly prevalent in the nineteenth and early twentieth centuries. The term assumed that humans could be clearly 'divided into distinct populations based on biological characteristics derived from their genetics, usually together with the belief that this also determined behaviour and institutions' (Littlewood, 1989b). As well as the arguments in relation to the colonial and derogatory nature of the term race, most contemporary authorities have argued that, as a biological notion, it is based on fallacious evidence and illogical arguments (Lévi-Strauss, 1985). It has however been retained by some communities and theorists as a sociological term – one which deals with a political world in which 'race' as a biologically descriptive term is still considered a valid term to understand culture and behaviour.

The word *culture* is generally taken to mean the 'total of non-biologically inherited patterns of shared experience and behaviour through which personal identity and social structures are attained in each generation in a particular society, whether ethnic group or a nation' (Littlewood, 1989b). It is seen as inter-subjective, as the process of transmitting conceptual and social guidelines to the next generation through the use of symbols, language, art and ritual (Helman, 1985). While such a definition identifies the dynamic nature of culture, this breadth of meaning and its apparent assumption of bounded and rigid groups has contributed to its current unpopularity as a descriptive term amongst many transcultural psychiatrists in Britain.

An *ethnic group* 'may be a nation, a people, a language group, a so-called race or a group bound together in a coherent cultural entity through a shared religion, belief in a common descent, or through the recognition of particular shared physical characteristics which are selected for remark or identity by the group or others' (Littlewood and Lipsedge, 1989). A *minority ethnic group* is a group which is 'dominated politically or numerically by larger (usually European) populations and social institutions. Such domination may be temporary or permanent, explicit or implicit' (Littlewood, 1989b).

Although such definitions seem quite precise, in practice assigning a person to a single ethnic or cultural group is often fraught with problems. This is a point I shall return to.

Migration and mental health

Although recent immigration laws have meant that fewer people are immigrating into Britain than previously (EEC migration excepted), it is important to reflect on some of the consequences of earlier migration. We find, for example, that some of the British-born children of migrants are still dealing with some of the unresolved experiences of *their* parents.

One of the first experiences that a migrant encounters is a variable degree of 'culture shock'. This is a phenomenon that most professionals broadly acknowledge, although there is disagreement as to its precise nature. The International Classification of Diseases, (WHO, 1978) includes it as a distinct category; the latest edition of the American Psychiatric Association's Diagnostic and Statistical Manual (the DSM-IIIR) does not provide a specific category, although it might be expected to be subsumed under 'adjustment disorder' (APA, 1987).

As with the continuing debate as to whether culture shock is a discrete entity, evidence of the effects of migration on people are highly contradictory. Furnham and Bochner (1986) describe one of the first studies that looked at the psychological consequences of migration. This was done in 1903 when the United States government carried out a census of all mental hospitals and found a greater than expected percentage of immigrants in these institutions (70% of the hospital population compared with 20% in the community). This led to argument as to whether immigrants should be allowed into the USA without first having checks made on their mental health, and later to the introduction of a screening procedure at Ellis Island. The data were re-evaluated by Malzberg in 1940. He found that if confounding variables were taken into account (those of gender, age, class, and marital status) then the proportion of immigrants in mental institutions dropped to 19% – about the same level as in the existing community.

Two rather different hypotheses have tried to explain how migration might have adverse psychological effects. The self-selection theory suggested that the migrants may either arrive in their new country with the illness already or were particularly vulnerable once they had settled. The social causation model suggested that the changes in life style, economics, family life, language and values might cause mental distress. (See Cochrane, 1983 for a fuller review.) Some studies have shown good adjustment in an immigrant population (Cochrane and Stopes-Roe, 1977), while a high rate of psychiatric morbidity in the children of migrants has been found by others (Harrison *et al*, 1988). Most studies fail to take into account the available social support structures for potential patients, their isolation from or geographical proximity to family and friends, their perceptions of illness and distress and their coping mechanisms, factors that are particularly relevant when we consider access to psychotherapy and counselling.

Full understanding of the stresses on any person involves an understanding of personal experience in the societies in which they were born and have lived, the effect of the transition from one country to another, the effects of being a migrant in a new country or the effects of living in a country where you were born but where that society still views you as 'an immigrant'.

Culture and self-identity

The UK 'ethnic minority population' can hardly be described as a migrant one. There is now a second, and often third generation which is British-born. While these people may have many of the same assumptions, lifestyle and experiences as their parents (as, for example, the experience of racism), the subtle differences of experience and response have yet to be studied (Acharyya *et al*, 1989).

We know from numerous studies that many minority ethnic groups continue to experience deprivation in the areas of housing, education, employment and health care, as well as sharing the experience of overt and covert racism in daily life (Littlewood and Lipsedge, 1989; Acharrya *et al.*, 1989). For the migrant generation itself, there is also the primary stress of dislocation and adjustment. Such experiences, if continued, are likely to have adverse psychological effects (Littlewood and Lipsedge, 1989).

From our study of clients coming to Nafsiyat, it is clear that a substantial minority of patients (23.1% in the prospective study) were British-born and whose parents or grandparents had migrated. This led us at an early stage to a dilemma. How should the professional/researcher allocate 'ethnicity' on the data sheets – in terms of the patients' place of birth or of their parents' or grandparents', or in terms of their self-perceived 'ethnic origin'? And what about those of mixed origin – how should they be allocated? Moreover, is this a relevant question to ask?

The following example (not the most complicated) attempts to highlight the researcher's quandary. This patient's parents came from India; she was born in East Africa and came to Britain at the age of two. Assigning her country of birth to Kenya seemed simple. Would this person however have had the same 'culture' or 'ethnicity' as an adult who had recently come to Britain from a similar background? Or one whose parents came from Bangladesh? She is a doctor: does this make her 'less Indian' than if she were a housewife? She is now married to 'an Indian' from the West Indies; what culture or ethnicity are her children born in Britain? From research at Nafsiyat we know that the term 'country of birth' on questionnaires can elicit a response that bears little relationship to the culture within which the client lives her or his life. In practice, professional agencies usually refer clients to us hoping for a therapist from the same background. This may be determined by where the patient was born or by the referring agent's perception of the client's culture. This may be as vague as 'Asian'.

Moreover, in looking at the referring professionals' dilemmas over determining ethnicity, it becomes evident that one of the most important issues presented by patients when confronting this issue would be in relation to their own 'identity'.

Variables in intercultural therapy

A major difficulty in psychotherapy research is that there are now many different types of therapy. Recently Karasu estimated that there were over four hundred relatively distinct types (1985). These range from the traditional psychoanalytic and other dynamic techniques, through client-centred therapies and cognitive therapy, to behavioural therapies. Some therapies use a group or family approach, others, an individual one. Some are directive, others not. More recently there has been research interest in the processes of therapeutic communities (Rosser *et al.*, 1987; Dolan *et al*, 1991). Comparison between studies is thus difficult. Even within distinct schools of therapy, technique varies between individual therapists; currently, in fact, we do not know how much the results from the different schools can be put together and generalised.

What is 'research'?

There are basic differences between those who believe that the efficacy of psychotherapy can and should be empirically evaluated (following Eysenck's (1952) challenge to psychotherapists to prove the worth of psychotherapy as compared with biomedical treatments), and those who do not believe it can be scientifically validated, and prefer simply descriptive or interpretative reports. Researchers in cross-cultural therapy have tended to concentrate their attention on specific identifiable aspects of the encounter, for example, differences in verbal/nonverbal communication, between therapists and client. Practising psychotherapists themselves have usually approached the question by presenting the results of their work in terms of detailed case reports, giving an account of the progress of a particular patient, the interaction between the two individuals, effects of particular interpretations and interventions, resolution of transference relationships, and so on. This may reflect not only the fact that most conventionally trained psychotherapists work in private practice and are unable to collect data on large populations, but also the attitudes and ideology of therapy itself as a 'humanistic', and thus arguably non-quantifiable, practice.

The uniqueness of intercultural work is, of course, one that specifies *difference*. Lago (1981) suggests that there are several possible types of cultural difference in therapy. There is the way in which emotional problems are presented to the counsellor (see also Rack, 1982) and the style of experiencing and communicating distress. There are also linguistic difficulties – not only those situations where the therapist speaks another language and communication is through an interpreter, but also those situations where literal translation of the patient's meanings may result in confusion for the counsellor (see also Marcos, 1988).

While some studies argue that there are universal patterns of non-verbal communication (Ekman and Friesen, 1971), others (Clark and Lago, 1980) suggest that this is not so. Other factors include the possible lack of awareness by the patient of what the offered therapy or counselling amounts to; failure by the counsellor to be aware of the patient's cultural and family constellation; and prejudicial attitudes (both conscious or unconscious) of both parties to each other. Although these headings are an oversimplification (and Lago admits that each incorporates several different problems) they do provide a framework within which we can begin to examine the issues that surround cross-cultural work.

In opposition to an emphasis on 'difference as problem', Patterson (1978) argues that cultural differences in counselling are of no greater import than class differences, and thus he suggests it would be equally valid to have specialised training for psychotherapists of the poor. In what Garfield and Bergin (1986) consider to be 'the most thorough review of the literature', Abramowitz and Murray (1983) found that white reviewers tended to minimise the effects of ethnicity, whilst black reviewers tended to emphasise findings in which differences are found.

Another issue raised in the cross-cultural field is that of the actual choice of appropriate therapy. Some authors support the use of group therapy as a way of overcoming the reticence and discomfort of black patients (see Bavington, Chapter 7, this volume). By contrast, Kanishige (1973) shows how contrary the egalitarian and unstructured procedures of group work are to the cultural values of many Asian Americans. Moreover, Harrison (1975) showed the existence of a general trend that people tend to prefer their counsellors to be of the same race.

Since the research at the Nafsiyat Centre looked at individual therapy, I shall confine my remarks to individual psychodynamic issues. Most individual psychotherapy can be described in terms of four prerequisites:

- It is an agreed contract between two people, the one with distress and the other with the training and expertise to alleviate that distress. Notable in such a relationship is the asymmetry of power relationship (which has particular resonances for cross-cultural work).
- It employs psychological processes and both verbal and nonverbal communication, within the therapeutic relationship.
- The psychotherapist deploys her concepts of transference and counter-transference to facilitate the treatment.
- The aim of therapy is to bring about relief, personality change and/or insight (see Draguns 1985; Bloch, 1982).

There are five obvious variables which psychotherapy research needs to be concerned with: the population studied, the types of distress presented, the therapist variables, the type of therapy employed, and the aims of the therapy.

(1) The population studied

This is particularly relevant for an intercultural therapy centre such as Nafsiyat. It is important that patients who have migrated are identified separately from those patients who are British born.

A recent British investigation of psychotherapy included the following as selection criteria: an absence of psychotic or obsessional characteristics, a continuous history of psychological disturbance of less than two years duration and current employment in a professional or managerial job (Shapiro *et al.*, 1989). This study broadly mirrors the selection criteria used by many practising psychotherapists. However, evidence suggests that problems may spontaneously remit within a two-year period (Eysenck, 1952) as the average duration of neurotic illness has been shown to be between one and two years (Shepherd and Wilkinson, 1988). What such a study may be measuring therefore as 'success' may include spontaneous remission rather than therapeutic efficacy.

Arguments have raged over several years about what 'spontaneous remission' rates actually mean. The assumption is usually that 'spontaneous' implies 'untreated'. However, spontaneous remission rates are likely to be affected by sharing one's problems with priests, a relative or even a friend. When considering the specificity of 'therapy' we are not talking of the effects of diffused psychotherapeutic processes which may occur in many, probably most, communities, so much as a specific additive procedure. The baseline of spontaneous remission may, however, be different for different ethnic groups.

(2) The distress

Eysenck states that 'researchers and therapists must define clearly and unambiguously what is meant by neurotic disorder and what is meant by cure; they must put forward methods of testing the effects of the treatment which are not dependent on subjective evaluations of the therapists, and they must demonstrate that their methods give results which are clearly superior to alternative methods such as those of behavioural therapy or of spontaneous remissions'. Most research thus far has not been able to meet these criteria.

Rachman and Wilson (1980) note that the evaluation of psychotherapy is generally confined to neurotic patients. They point out that there are three basic assumptions in all conventional outcome research. The first is that there is an implicit accommodation of psychological difficulties within a medical model: hence 'neurotic'. Secondly, there is an assumption that a key symptom, anxiety, is a unitary concept and a universal experience; they note that Lang (1969) has argued persuasively for a more complex conception in which 'anxiety' can be seen as a set of at least three loosely coupled components – verbal reports, behavioural avoidance, and psychophysiological changes – which has implications for the design of research. The third assumption is that while setting up their own measures of therapeutic change (such as therapists' impressions, patients' expressions of satisfaction, changed scores on personality tests, etc.), they have adopted rather soft signs of change.

To the above list I would add that there is a fourth assumption: that whoever carries out the therapy (whether trained or not) is actually facilitating change through psychotherapy, and a fifth, that all psychotherapy is addressing the same kind of problems (e.g. 'neurotic' problems). Medical anthropology has, however, reminded us that conceptions of distress, and their communication, are social in origin, specific to particular groups and situations, and thus unlikely to be similar in different groups, and not easily translated into some unitary medical schema which can then be compared across cultures (see Littlewood, 1990).

(3) Therapist variables

In many of the existing studies there has not been sufficient explanation of the actual style of therapy offered. Although a therapist may have been trained in a particular school, there are always adaptations in technique with different patients; the differences between radical and less radical departures need, therefore, to be assessed. Such departures may be particularly likely when a therapist responds to the presenting patterns of a patient of a different culture.

Other therapist variables include attitudes and beliefs of the therapist regarding the types of patient to be taken on, the number of previous patients treated, length of time since training or whether still in training, and experience of training analysis. Although all of these do have implications for the quality of the therapy given, it is obviously difficult to closely match therapists in any particular study. It would seem sensible, therefore, to record such information and replace the current situation where therapists are simply described as 'experienced', 'inexperienced' or 'in training'. Additionally, we need to examine the type of cultural difference between therapist and patient, and whether the former has previous experience of intercultural work.

It has been noted in many studies that therapists tend to select patients who are young, attractive, verbal, intelligent and successful (the so-called YAVIS effect). How many black patients, however young, are likely to be perceived by white therapists as attractive, verbal, intelligent or successful? There have been few large-scale evaluations of psychotherapy, the most notable being the 15-year Menninger Clinic study (Kernberg *et al.*, 1972). This devised its own measures of client attributes which suggested the patients who did well in psychotherapy were those with good initial ego strength, high initial quality of interpersonal relationships, high initial anxiety tolerance, and high motivation. Again we have to consider any racial bias in such therapists' interpretation of these criteria and whether such criteria are comparable with those of other studies.

Ironically, some of the best evidence that psychotherapy 'works' comes from studies of behaviour therapy, where psychotherapy has been used as a control (Rachman and Wilson, 1980). It is interesting to note that in most of these studies the 'therapist' was untrained or in training – it might be expected then that if therapy works it will be the trained and experienced therapists who achieve the best results. This poses the question whether better results would have been achieved with well trained, experienced therapists.

Luborsky *et al.*, (1975), found that in most studies it was the therapist who was the most common means of assessment: the majority of their patients are seen by them as making slight to moderate gains. Feifil and Eells (1963), however, found important differences in emphasis between the reports of the patients and those of their therapists: the therapists giving greater importance to insight and technique while patients rated self-understanding and self-confidence as important. Given the inevitable bias, we need to use 'independent' measures of well-being, and then see how these correspond with the opinions of both therapist and patient. Clearly, everybody wants their patients to do well, a factor we have to take into account in the area of intercultural work where so much seems to rest on the question 'does it work?'.

(4) Type of therapy employed

As we noted above, there are hundreds of 'different' types of therapy. Many therapists now work eclectically, using the therapeutic tools of more than one school of thought. This needs to be identified in any research. Do the modalities of different therapists converge in their intercultural work? Is the difference in commitment to intercultural work such that previous training is less significant in comparing different therapeutic styles?

(5) The aims of the therapy

The definition of the aims of psychotherapy is, of course, intrinsic to the way the therapy is evaluated by practitioners. Some critics (Rachman and Wilson, 1980) have argued that we need to replace the usual medical definitions of personal problems with psychological definitions, assessed by psychological methods. Such changes, they state, would involve a departure from conventional concepts of cure, relapse and prognosis.

For some studies, the aims are simply symptom removal (a medical model), while for others it is some type of rebuilding of the personality (a psychoanalytic model). Others have argued for the middle ground (as in the short-term psychotherapies advocated by Malan [1975]).

The goals of therapy, and thus its evaluation, present special problems for patients and therapists of different cultures. Who defines such a thing as an 'acceptable change in personality'? Do minority patients simply want the removal of distressing symptoms as many psychotherapists argue? Does psychotherapy anyway change the personality, or merely reframe presenting difficulties? Pederson (1981) considers these differences in relation to the conventional distinction between 'emic' understanding, which is the understanding of a culture in its own terms, and the 'etic' approach which attempts to consider cultural and personal factors in some sort of general pan-cultural theory, whether biological, psychological or social.

Can we combine the two? Kareem (1987) argues that intercultural therapy is a therapy that 'takes into account the whole being of the patient – not only the individual concepts and constructs as presented to the therapist, but also the patients' communal life experience in the world – both past and present. The very fact of being from another culture employs both conscious and unconscious assumptions – both in the patient and in the therapist; and we believe that for the successful outcome of therapy, addressing these assumptions is essential'. If this is our goal, evaluation has to include measures which make sense in terms of our clients' own understandings, as well as those applicable to some idea of a valid identity, and more universal measures of personal life within the social world.

Research at Nafsiyat

Research at the Centre was set up against a committed background of trying to understand why ethnic minorities were not considered appropriate referrals to psychotherapy centres. Which groups would use a psychotherapy centre that dealt with issues of 'culture'? To what extent could people from ethnic and cultural minority backgrounds be helped by psychotherapy?

From its inception we had felt it was important to monitor the work of the Centre. The research programme that was set up therefore comprised three stages: a retrospective study, questionnaire development, and a prospective study.

The retrospective study

This study evaluated the population seen at the Centre on referral as well as socio-demographic data. Since the Centre began in 1983, 346 patients had been referred. The data collection was begun in 1986. One in three cases was screened, using a quasi-random sampling technique. Of these, only those assessed and treated by the Clinical Director were analysed in detail (54 cases).

Results suggested that using a 'project diagnosis' of each patient's problem (following DSM-III criteria), 13% of the patients could be described as having symptoms suggestive of schizophrenia, paranoid psychosis or the major affective disorders. Moreover, 13% were being referred to the Centre with these symptoms. (These were not all the same patients; in some cases the referral diagnosis and the Nafsiyat Centre diagnosis were different.)

It was also found that the patients had been seeking help from other medical/psychiatric professionals over a period of time. The other major finding was the diversity of backgrounds of the patients: 22 different countries of birth were identified. Of these, the largest group were the British born. The peak age range for referrals was the 20–35 age range; the sex ratio was 3:2 females:males. There were high levels of self referral with over one-third of patients being referred this way.

The major limitation of this study, as it was a retrospective analysis, was that we had no 'objective' measures of psychological distress before and after treatment.

The prospective study

This part of the research comprised two groups. We continued the general assessment with a total referred group who comprised 157 consecutive patients who were assessed in terms of demographic and referral variables. A random subset of the 157 – a treatment group of 52 patients – were assessed before and after therapy using the General Health Questionnaire (Goldberg et al., 1978) and the Present State Examination (Wing et al., 1974).

New questionnaires, developed at the Centre, were used to collect case history and social history information. Each therapist completed a psychiatric checklist, a therapy action schedule, and a therapy profile; patients were asked to fill out a feedback form.

When the results were evaluated it was found that the treatment group were similar to the referred group in terms of sex ratio (2.3 compared with 1.7), origin in North London (65% and 66%), self-referral (58% compared to 62%), general practitioner referral (21% compared to 19%), and psychiatric referral (11% and 9%). Men were more likely to be referred (by doctors) than women. Few patients from either group had requested a therapist of a particular ethnic origin. The major origins of the patients in the referred group were one-quarter UK, one-fifth West Indies, one-sixth Africa, one-sixth South Asia (the treatment group were similar except that only one-tenth were born in Africa).

In the treatment group a high proportion had completed secondary education; nine were unemployed. Over half the group were living in council or housing trust accommodation. Of the total, 85% were not paying for their therapy.

The most common presenting problems were depression and a general 'inability to cope'; a number of patients presented with 'identity problems'. Of the women, 25% reported rape or other sexual abuse.

In 46% the therapy was short term – 15 sessions or less – and was focused on a specific event. In 42% of the 52 cases the therapy was one contract (i.e. 12 sessions) or less. In 25% of cases the therapy was long term but focused on a particular issue while in almost 30% of patients the therapy was long term and looked more at changing adaptive styles and coping. Of the treatment group, 73% had not been offered psychotherapy previously.

Only in very rare cases were patients seen more regularly than once a week, usually to help them over a crisis period. Moreover, the majority of long-term patients in the study came for under one year of therapy, although 12% had been seeking help for their problem for over five years.

At the end of therapy, two questions were asked to see whether the patients themselves felt they had benefited: (1) had they found the therapy useful? (2) would they recommend it to a friend with similar problems? Of those who replied, 91% said that they had found the therapy useful and would recommend it to a friend.

The 60-item General Health Questionnaire (GHQ) was used to measure change. It is a self-report inventory which distinguishes between those not psychiatrically ill (who score less than 12), those who are currently having problems but who will get better without treatment (who score 12–19), and those who need psychiatric intervention (a score of 20+), (Johnstone and Goldberg, 1976). There are several problems with the scale, notably the cut off score chosen for each section when the questionnaire is used with a non-white British population. Some authors have argued for different scores for different ethnic populations (e.g. Harding, 1976; Lattanzi *et al.*, 1988; Kitamura *et al.*, 1989), while others have claimed this reduces the sensitivity of the instrument (Vasquez-Barquero *et al.*, 1986). However, in a multi-ethnic situation, with patients of such diverse backgrounds, it was considered appropriate to retain Goldberg's original scoring, and to compare the results with the Present State Examination (PSE).

The second major problem was that the questionnaire asks the patient to answer the questions in relation to how they had been feeling over the last three weeks: for people who have chronic illnesses there may have been no change over the last few weeks so they would respond using 'the same as usual' response. This response scores zero and thus does not count towards the final 'illness score'. Hence the initial GHQ may be an underestimate of the level of distress (but see Goodchild and Duncan-Jones, 1985 and Koeter *et al.*, 1989). The PSE was therefore used as a comparative measure.

In spite of these reservations, the GHQ can be taken as some measure of what is a case, i.e. of psychiatric 'caseness'. A common challenge to workers in this area is that concepts of psychotherapy might be better adapted to people from one ethnic minority than other ethnic minorities. However, a comparison of the initial and final GHQ scores found no evidence to suggest

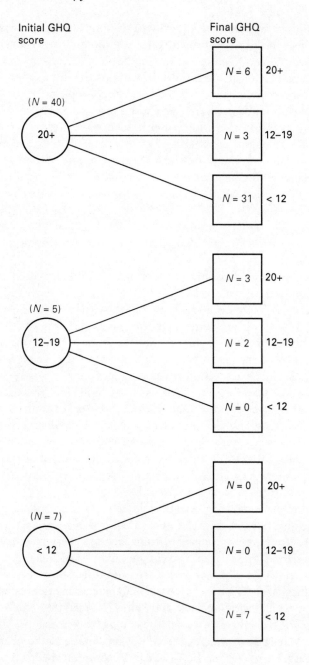

Fig. 6.1 Changes in number of patients in each GHQ group – before and after therapy.

any relationship between the ethnicity of the client and the scores before or after therapy or the degree of change. (There was a non-statistically significant relationship between final GHQ and ethnic origin when the initial GHQ score was over 20.) There was no relationship between initial or final GHQ and either age or sex.

Only seven patients had GHQ scores indicating 'no symptomatology'. Of the 40 patients with initial GHQ scores in the high range (conventionally thought not to resolve spontaneously), six remained in this category after treatment. Figures 6.1 and 6.2 illustrate these results.

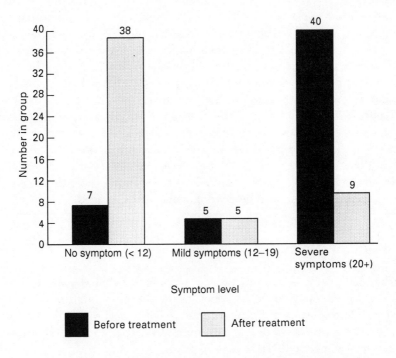

Fig. 6.2 General Health Questionnaire: results before and after therapy.

Using the PSE, initial measures before treatment suggested quite a high degree of severe psychiatric distress: 19% of the treatment group had Catego categories corresponding to schizophrenia, hypomania and 'non-specific psychosis'. A total of 42 patients had the Syndrome Checklist (SCL) category of simple depression and 46 had other SCL depressive syndromes.

Obviously, we cannot claim these results as any sort of conclusive proof of the efficacy of the treatment. Further research needs to be done with larger numbers of different ethnic groups, and of patients with similar patterns of symptoms, so that a clearer picture can be built up of any relations between ethnicity and outcome, and between distress and outcome.

The study only examined 'inputs' and 'outputs'. How specific is the therapy? What are the characteristics which make it work? What is the significance of the feeling of 'safety' that the clients frequently report: is it because the Nafsiyat Centre is seen as a place for therapy for black people or is it merely that the Centre itself is not part of the hospital system?

As the majority of clients do not pay for their therapy, it is difficult to compare outcomes for paying and non-paying clients. As the Centre has a fair 'success' rate, however, it suggests that payment in itself is not necessary for motivation. Most of the patients would not have been able to attend if cost effective payment had been required. Some of the patients were unemployed (some having lost jobs through their symptoms), several were students, and a few were single parents or in especially low paid jobs. Only 30 of the 52 were in full-time employment. Another way of identifying those with limited finances is to look at the type of housing they occupy: A total of 48% lived in Council accommodation with the private rented sector accounting for only three patients; just over 30% lived in their own accommodation or shared a mortgage; four people had Housing Trust accommodation.

If the Centre took on only those from a professional or managerial background, or who were financially secure, clearly most of the patients whose cases are described here would have been excluded.

Conclusions

What do these results mean? I would suggest that they show that the view that black and ethnic minority people cannot benefit from formal therapy is wrong. The research also suggests, albeit with small numbers, that people who show severe symptoms as determined by conventional rating scales may benefit from psychotherapy.

Our continuing research is concerned with devising a schema that can show how different therapist training influences the therapeutic technique eventually employed. At the same time, we try to avoid the simplistic data collection assumptions that can trap the unwary.

Future research also needs to consider the problem of assessing 'ethnicity' so that a person's background and values are more meaningfully identified. We need to compare the effectiveness of the different approaches with different presenting problems. Individual patient variables are also likely to play an important role. Currently we are carrying out multivariate analysis in order to elicit the particular complex of factors that determine good or poor outcome.

Part III: Practice

Chapter 7

The Bradford Experience

JOHN BAVINGTON

The industrial city of Bradford has a long history of immigration dating back to the last century when it was known as the 'wool capital of the world', with a textile industry which attracted many migrant workers. In the post-war years these included groups from Eastern Europe (mostly Polish but also from the Ukraine, Latvia, Lithuania, Estonia, Hungary and Yugoslavia) and in the 1950s, workers were recruited from the Indian subcontinent and from the Caribbean. Initially the majority were younger men but since then wives and families have come over in increasing numbers. There are now large settled communities of black and ethnic minorities amounting to about 20% of Bradford's population of half a million.

These include South Asians from mainly rural areas of Kashmir, especially Mirpur, and Bangladeshis from Sylhet, Sikhs from the Punjab, and a small number of Gujarati-speaking Hindus from East Africa and elsewhere. Such a cultural diversity obviously includes a variety of languages, backgrounds, religions, and differing levels of formal education and literacy. Many people continue to keep in close contact with their places of origin, and there is much coming and going within the tight restrictions imposed by the present immigration regulations. A small number of the earliest, and now elderly, immigrants have returned or would like to return to their country of origin, but most consider they will now remain in the UK, as British citizens.

The transcultural unit

Lynfield Mount Hospital in Bradford opened in 1967 to deliver comprehensive psychiatric services to the central area of Bradford. It soon became clear that the needs of local ethnic minorities were being inadequately met, and Philip Rack, one of the three consultant psychiatrists, convened a multidisci-

Table 7.1 The Intercultural Team at Lynfield Mount Hospital (1990).

Discipline	Gender	Background	Minority language spoken
Consultant Psychiatrist	M	England/Pakistan	Urdu/Pushtu
Registrar/SHO	M	England/India	Punjabi
Clinical Assistant	M	India	Tamil/Telegu Hindi/Bengali (Malayalam)
Clinical Assistant	F	India	Bengali/Hindi
Senior Registrar	M	Holland	Dutch
Community Nurse	M	Mauritius	French/Hindi
Ward OT	F	England	—
Secretary to Consultant/Team	F	England/India	Punjabi
Communications Assistant	F	India	Urdu/Gujarati
Social Worker	F	India	Mahrati/Gujarati Hindi
Social Worker	M	Poland	Polish/German
Social Work Aide	F	India	Bengali/Hindi Punjabi
Senior Clinical Psychologist	F	Hungary	Hungarian
Art Therapist	F	England/Uganda	—
Team Leader in Social Work	F	Poland	Polish/German Russian
Principal Clinical Psychologist	M	England	—
Hospital Chaplain	M	Nigeria	Yoruba
Researcher	M	England	—
Senior Registrar	F	England	—

plinary group so that 'all patients referred to the hospital should be treated by this team if linguistic, cultural or adaptational problems seemed to be significant factors' (Rack, 1982).

The numbers of both patients and staff grew steadily and the group began to acquire some degree of experience and skill through daily clinical work and collective reflection and discussion. It is currently composed of 19 individuals in designated posts from various disciplines, ethnic (and therefore linguistic), and cultural backgrounds (Table 7.1). Ward nursing staff are also involved when possible. Apart from the Social Work Assistant, Communication Assistant and Consultant Psychiatrist, most members give only a small part of their time to the team.

Transcultural issues – out-patients

In trying to identify areas of difficulty in working with minority groups, and apart from the obvious one of language, we have defined two other overlapping areas (adapted from our handbook of services): those of cultural background and stress. 'The presentation and symptomatology of mental illness is not identical in all cultures; the means by which people signal distress are culturally grounded. It may therefore be difficult to decide whether a particular behaviour or complaint is a sign of mental illness or not. The dynamics of social and domestic stress, which may be associated with mental disturbance, can only be understood in their cultural context. In order to avoid errors, such "cultural awareness" is essential in approaching any patient/client whose background differs from the professional's own. It is our opinion that for really effective intervention, therefore, it is necessary that the professional be thoroughly acquainted with the patient's/client's particular cultural background.

'Members of minority ethnic groups in Britain are subject to particular stresses. These include socio-economic deprivation, racial discrimination, cultural alienation and numerous other sources of conflict, both between groups and within any one group. No accurate assessment of a person's mental health is possible without a detailed knowledge of the ways in which these stresses may impinge on the person's functioning in a concrete, day-to-day sense.'

The post of 'Communications Assistant' arose because of a realisation of inadequacies on the in-patient ward. It was decided to provide a post with a better status, salary, job description (hence the choice of a different title) and prospects than the usual interpreting arrangements made within the National Health Service. The post required some training and experience in the skills of interpreting such as that provided by the Bradford College's ABLE course (Access to Bilingual Employment). It was envisaged that the person would be available in a variety of situations in addition to those of the ward, be responsible for translation of written materials and also act as the administrator for the team. The person appointed has not only provided a high level of purely linguistic interpretation but has also acquired the role of patients' advocate. She has also enhanced her abilities by taking counselling training, and now has a therapeutic role, working especially with families and in establishing patient groups. It has been one of the most imaginative and constructive steps in our growth and we would recommend it as a model.

Over the ten years of the writer's association with the Unit, some shift of emphasis and perspective can be detected. There have been changes of diagnostic practice but also more awareness of the common shared experience of social stress – especially in the South Asian communities. This knowledge has been supplemented by the recognition of vulnerability related to emotional disturbance in the countries of origin: for example, the finding that the oldest child of a family is liable to depression, especially if the parent of the same sex dies early. Similarly, it is possible to identify protective factors, resources and strengths within the community or family. A frequent element in illness experiences after migration has been the weakening of the network of family support with increasing distance, and the subsequent difficulties for the family in responding in the usual way when problems arise (Bavington, 1982). The team has also become more sensitive to the socio-economic deprivation of the minorities, the often hidden but all-pervading racist attitudes within our institutions, and the experience of this by our patients which weighs down their morale and self-esteem, is sometimes felt acutely, painfully and bitterly, leading directly to some form of emotional disturbance.

In terms of day-to-day organisation, out-patient clinics are held at least one morning a week on a day when most members of the team are able to get together. Clinics are mainly run by the medical members of the team and are similar to other clinics in the hospital rather than seen as separate 'transcultural clinics'. Their distinctiveness lies in the fact that almost every patient will be seen by someone able to talk the same language. This means that they can be seen in the first place on their own without the need to use relatives as interpreters (although close relatives are frequently involved at some later stage). Social work and other expertise can be called upon when needed, and the regular nursing staff of the out-patient department, while not members of the transcultural unit, have gained considerable experience through their contacts with our team and patients.

Two group meetings are also held, one for mainly Polish clients, the other a mixed Asian group in Urdu/Punjabi. Most practical and administrative matters are dealt with here but, more importantly, these meetings provide the main opportunity for wider discussion on many of the issues relevant to intercultural work: 'an ongoing exercise in mutual education from which everyone benefits, the indigenous English member probably most of all' (Rack, 1982).

As part of the wider learning programme the Unit has also for many years set aside time every month for a larger open meeting to which various local professionals are invited. This usually takes the form of a particular guest speaker dealing with some matter of interest, not necessarily psychiatric, and can attract an audience of 70, including local health visitors, social workers, community workers, GPs and other physicians. Increasingly also there are requests from students, trainees or others who wish to see something of our work. Recent examples include a teacher of deaf Asian children; a film maker producing videos to publicise the local Social Security provisions in several Asian languages; a lecturer in sociology; two workers starting an Asian Women's Centre in Leeds; someone planning the production of written materials on Mental Health matters for patients in different languages; and a local community group bringing samples of Asian meals for us to 'test'.

Since our primary clinical responsibility is to a population of perhaps 50 000, some team members are available on a daily basis to cover the usual range of services such as visits to homes or other hospitals. In addition, the team is further developing its community psychiatry links with primary services and community agencies and is able to take a number of referrals from neighbouring districts or further afield.

Transcultural issues – in-patients

Although patients needing admission form a relatively small proportion (an average at any time of 6–7 in-patients), they are usually the most distressed. They often feel helpless and at the mercy of others, and for a few, these will be compulsory admissions under the Mental Health Act. Particular consideration must be given to the needs of this group, and the ward organisation, facilities and staff all need to be appropriate.

Probably the most useful development at Lynfield Mount Hospital, has been the employment of some staff who are themselves from a South Asian background and who are able to speak the most commonly needed languages. At present the nursing staff includes one Mauritian, two Pakistanis and two white nurses who are learning Urdu. In addition, we have found that when someone learns another language they nearly always acquire with it other important attributes, including enhanced sensitivity and cultural knowledge. While white nurses have learned much of value over years of contact with minority patients, it is only recently that any detailed thought has been given to recruitment procedures for all nurses, including the requirement of a special interest, experience or qualifications for the multi-ethnic composition of the hospital's population.

Regular group therapy in Punjabi and Urdu occurs as part of the therapeutic programme and there are regular community meetings, open to any members of the staff or patients. General issues concerning the use of groups across culture are discussed elsewhere in this volume; as regards the situation at Lynfield Mount, particularly with regard to South Asian patients who are a small minority in unfamiliar surroundings, they face strange and unsettling conditions of a mixed ward (with no proper *purdah* area); thus, the group meeting is regarded as a haven and tends to develop group cohesion much more rapidly than other groups, with lively interaction and visible concern for others. The group has, on occasion, been able to request improvements in our facilities, such as more appropriate dietary provisions (Bavington, 1989) and the need for a secluded area for women.

Specific approaches to therapy

Much of the day-to-day care of patients who are referred to the out-patient clinics is similar to that offered to indigenous white patients; it has to be remembered, however, that just as experience and clinical presentation of illness are influenced by medical views, beliefs and context, the expectations of the patient and family too are important: they may be unfamiliar with medical notions of 'psychological illness'. Patients referred are often unhappy at having to come to a psychiatric hospital, feeling that it implies that they are 'mad'. Mahendra Dayal (1987), from his work in Birmingham, describes a similar reaction: 'The clients' initial behaviour is influenced by their own preconceived ideas about the hospital and helping agency, family attitudes towards mental illness, a sense of loss of prestige and status amongst relatives and friends, and long-term repercussions within the larger family and community at large. Being mentally ill may be construed as a blot on the family honour and prestige, affecting the long-term future prospects of children regarding their engagements, marriages, etc.'

Often patients are not given an adequate explanation of the referral beyond being told they are to see a 'specialist'. Thus, their initial presentation and expectation has to do with hope of receiving some physical investigation (especially an X-ray of the head) and some form of medication. On the other hand 'ideas about the potential dangers of Western medicine (often considered by Asians as "hot" and hence potentially harmful) or the value of injection, or information on the significance of timing and diet in relation to the taking of drugs are important' (Bavington and Majid, 1986). As Dayal

(1987) notes, 'An Asian client does not see any importance or relevance of family matters, relationship conflicts, inter- and intra-familial stresses, to their personal suffering. GPs and many workers are well aware of such a client's stereotyped presentation of various somatic symptoms, grudging acceptance and lack of compliance about drugs, and increasing demand of various physical illness. They often show a tremendous fear of being hooked on drugs and adamantly resist any suggestion of psychological problems or relationship difficulties'.

Such fears are only confirmed if they are then prescribed the standard doses of psychiatric drugs – these do indeed cause many side effects since it has now been fairly well established that a satisfactory therapeutic response can be obtained with lower doses (especially in the case of antidepressant drugs), than are traditionally used in Western countries. This appears to be confirmed by research findings that higher blood levels are achieved in African or Asian than white subjects after the same dose of antidepressant. It is the experience of the Transcultural Unit that appropriate medication has an important part to play – depending, of course, on the diagnosis. There have been instances of schizophrenia being misdiagnosed in patients who when correctly treated have made good progress and remained almost symptom-free. Perhaps our largest group are those suffering from varying degrees of depression and anxiety. Many of these may require some initial antidepressant medication and are very disappointed and disillusioned if no such help is offered. While it may be argued that this is likely to reinforce the 'medical model' and the patient's view of themselves as being physically ill, this has generally not been found to be the case; rather, I have found that providing a medicine is a step towards establishing common ground for other forms of therapy.

Therapeutic approaches

Psychotherapy itself has been a rather inadequately covered aspect of our services in Bradford. The team still has no fully trained and qualified psychotherapist. An even greater obstacle has been perhaps the questioning and debate over the applicability of such approaches across cultures. There is the often repeated assertion that psychotherapies, as practised in Britain, 'have their roots in the Western world and were devised, developed, and formulated on the basis of a Western philosophy of life which in many respects contradicts the traditional beliefs and ideology of those who have come from other parts of the world and have different religious and value systems' (Bavington and Majid, 1986).

In my view, the appropriate response is not to discount altogether the value of such methods, but to consider what might constitute a more relevant and acceptable form of psychotherapy. Such an approach would evolve a synthesis that incorporated elements of the existing methods, some of which may in any case be fairly universal, while also recognising basic concepts from the other culture. Dayal (1987) suggests a cross-cultural approach: 'Concepts originating in one culture are adapted and translated into the ideas, practices and language of the other. The relative contribution by each culture is more towards the relationship which is mutually adaptive and brings a closer fit'. This is an area where much work still needs to be done.

There are certain elements or basic principles of psychotherapy which can be regarded as relatively universal and culture free (Chapter 3). Take, for example, the definition offered by Brown and Pedder: 'Psychotherapy is essentially a conversation which involves listening to and talking with those in trouble with the aim of helping them understand and resolve their predicament' (Brown and Pedder, 1980). Such a statement would probably be acceptable across cultures and apply to a wide variety of help-giving relationships in varied settings and with quite diverse assumptions, except perhaps for the final part concerning 'understanding and resolving of predicaments'. It is mainly in the detailed working out in the therapeutic conversation that issues of 'culture' may arise. For example, while the general aim may well be to 'help', there may be differences or uncertainty on both sides as to what form the help should take. It has often been our experience that what is initially sought is very different from what later emerges, that this initial presentation certainly has to be accepted if any progress is to be made. There then follows a process of negotiation which may include making concessions and finding common ground as a way of establishing therapeutic alliance.

It has been our frequent experience that patients certainly acknowledge and recognise the value of such a 'conversation' but only up to a point: 'Thank you for this talk doctor, it was very interesting – now what about the treatment?' Patients often quote a common Urdu saying that, 'the doctor's *ikhlaq* [benevolence, or kindness] is half the treatment'. This again may be taken as some implicit appreciation of the value of a psychotherapeutic relationship, but this statement is frequently followed by a demand for the other half! Response to this may involve something more directive such as the prescription of a drug or some guidance on relaxation techniques, by, for example, supplying a relaxation cassette (one has recently been prepared in Urdu). One value of having a team of varied background is that it allows greater flexibility in finding the best match between client and therapist. But it is not always clear what is in fact 'best'.

Sometimes it seems obvious that both client and therapist should be from a similar background. A white therapist and a black patient (or vice versa) may certainly face additional obstacles but, if handled with awareness of the effects of racist attitudes, they may in fact facilitate the facing of certain matters when these are important for the therapy. Indeed, there is often therapeutic value in some degree of cultural distance. The 'inverse square law' put forward by Rack (1982) that 'empathy diminishes as the square of the cultural distance' may not always apply. The very ignorance of the therapist can be used to strengthen the patient's autonomy: 'what would you usually do in this situation according to your own family values?' The unfamiliarity of the situation may help to prise someone loose from inappropriate assumptions. It is also worth remembering that psychotherapy in some ways is always 'counter-cultural' in that it means examining and confronting shared implicit factors which may contribute to conflict and illness. The therapeutic situation itself allows the individual to step outside their usual taken-for-granted framework and to obtain a kind of freedom (and respon-sibility) not possible when enmeshed in the usual conventions of society.

Doubt has often been expressed as to the applicability of group therapy in the Asian context. The reasons given include linguistic difficulties, lack of 'psychological mindedness' and a reluctance to 'open up' in a group situation. However, our group in Bradford began eight years ago and has been described in detail by Das (1986), one of the team involved in the early days of its development. Its initial membership was a handful of Asian patients from the Lynfield Mount Hospital and the adjacent day hospital. Much of its initial impetus came from a long-standing English male member of the team, the local community relations chaplain, who became the group facilitator.

He was later joined by a female Indian social worker, and an Asian female trainee psychiatrist. At first, 'many of the patients were frightened and nervous about joining the group because they had no idea what it was all about; they were acutely embarrassed about discussing problems in front of strangers . . . . These patients were reassured repeatedly and given, as in the case of all patients, the option to leave the group at any time they found it distressing. The idea of discussing and sharing their distress with others who were experiencing similar problems was also discussed. The social worker was usually successful in obtaining their co-operation and it was surprising how nearly all of them looked forward to attending the group after their first meeting' (Das, 1986).

The chaplain, as a 'representative white' sometimes found himself the subject of feelings related to members' experiences of racism. Initially, there was a strong tendency to focus on 'the doctor' with direct medical questions. Similarly, the Indian social worker would be under pressure to provide help and advice on social and financial matters. With time, however, and as a result of clarification of the roles of the therapist, change occurred.

In terms of group interaction, 'once the members had accepted that she was not there as a "doctor" a phase of group evaluation of the therapist started. She was asked questions about her origins, religion, marital status, number of children, where she was educated, whether she had in-laws, had she lived with them, etc., etc. – in short, she was asked "Did she share their customs and values?" and "Was she capable of understanding their emotions?" . . . . Reassured that she shared their cultural background, was aware of the social and family issues and the meaning of certain behaviour, the conversation spontaneously became psychologically orientated. Regular members encouraged the newer members to discuss their emotional problems and gave them support, advice and hope. Conflict about "loss of role", "depression", "delusions", "mental illness", "religious differences" and "behavioural problems" were discussed freely and openly. It was obvious that once the members knew what the actual purpose of the group was and how they could be helped by it, they were prepared to use it to maximum advantage with the therapist acting as facilitator.' (Das).

This experience has now been replicated with several other groups and has convinced our own group that group therapy is not only possible but that it has great potential. The writer, while working previously in Pakistan, found mixed, daily in-patient groups to be acceptable in conservative Peshawar where they came to be known as 'the family meeting'. Here, 'It was found that the richer concept of the family was a useful way to evoke caring responses in the group' (Bavington, 1982).

Whatever may be the dynamics of the 'somatisation' process, the comments of Nasir Ilahi (Ilahi, 1989), a psychotherapist working in Southall, have been amply confirmed: 'Indians show a high level of intuitive awareness of the links between the emotional stresses of extended family living and somatic problems, especially in women'. Das, too, comments: 'There is a dynamic interaction and clients express their understanding and feelings about their own psychiatric problems and that of fellow members eloquently. Clients themselves have expressed their reasons for "somatisation"' (Das, 1986, personal communication).

The future

Currently, since the retirement of Philip Rack, much consideration is being given as to how best the transcultural work could relate to the hospital's own policy of moving more into the community; this has resulted in a breaking down of its 'catchment area' into several smaller sectors, each being served by a multidisciplinary psychiatric team based at a local Mental Health Centre. Such a move undoubtedly favours more awareness of and contact with the local population groups as each Mental Health Centre's brief includes planning and providing services according to these locally identified needs. In the future it is envisaged that most patients, including those from ethnic minority groups, will in the first place be seen away from the hospital, and that there will be closer work with primary health care, social work and other agencies. This will require changes in the structure of the Transcultural Unit's operations with, it is to be hoped, a greater input into all aspects of the local mental health services. It should provide greater opportunities for contact with various community organisations so that the service providers become more aware of the issues and needs as perceived by the users themselves, and more open to new ideas and to modifications of the existing patterns of health care delivery.

Chapter 8

Familiar and Unfamiliar Types of Family Structure: Towards a Conceptual Framework

ROSINE JOZEF PERELBERG

Family therapists have become increasingly concerned with the identification of patterns underlying communications within the family (Minuchin *et al.*, 1967). The term 'pattern', which the Concise Oxford Dictionary defines as 'regular form or order', implies the notions of shape and repetition (Cooklin, 1982). It suggests that when a group of people – such as a family – interact face to face, their interaction is made up of regularly repeated sequences whose form is relatively stable. These sequences, observable during family therapy sessions, are considered to be both events in themselves and also to express the major characteristics of interactions between the family members in other contexts of family life.

In their concern with patterns of relationships, family therapists have increasingly focused on the behavioural and emotional properties of relationships (Gorrell Barnes, 1982). At the behavioural level, the therapist looks at the sequence of actions that can be identified at a descriptive level, i.e. who talks to whom and at what moment during the session, who interrupts whom, who does not speak unless specifically invited to do so, and so on. At the emotional level it is the mood or affect in the session that is characterised. Thus, a family can appear 'happy', 'angry', 'flat', 'friendly', 'hostile', etc. This assessment presupposes the existence of empathy between the observer and the family insofar as the former is able to identify the family's mood.

This chapter sets out to suggest that it is only by considering the meaning of patterns of interaction that the 'family map' can be identified. An understanding at this level requires the therapist to pay attention to the ways in which family members themselves understand their behaviour. This level of meaning is present in all encounters between therapists and families but it is only in certain contexts that the therapist is made aware of its existence.

I hope here to develop the concept of family map to indicate the way in which it differs from, and relates to, that of culture. I will then outline a conceptual framework which connects the concepts of 'culture', 'family map', and 'patterns of interaction', and consider its conceptual and clinical implications for family therapy.

Culture and ethnicity

Most of the family therapy literature which has considered the cultural context in which families are placed has resulted from work with 'ethnic families' (e.g. McGoldrick *et al.*, 1982; Falicov and Carter, 1980; Herz, 1982; Kaslow, 1982 and Foley, 1982). The most important result of this body of work has been the creation of background material relating to the range and diversity of ethnic groups in the USA. The fact that this interest in the notion of culture stems from work with 'exotic' families involves the implicit danger of associating culture with that which is unfamiliar. In contrast, what one is familiar with is 'naturalised' and thus perceived of as part of 'nature'.

Since most of this work is largely descriptive, it does not raise the question of a conceptual framework in terms of which families can be understood. Categories of 'ethnicity' and 'culture' are used interchangeably. To take one example: 'Ethnicity patterns our thinking, feeling and behaviour in both obvious and subtle ways' and 'our cultural values and assumptions are generally outside our awareness' (McGoldrick, 1982: p. 4).

The notion of culture itself is mostly perceived in general terms, as if cultures were monolithic entities sometimes defined with geographic boundaries, e.g. the Irish, the Germans, the Italians (Ablon, 1980), the Asians (Shon and Ja, 1982), the British (McGill and Pearce, 1982), and the Italians (Rotunno and McGoldrick, 1982). Internal differentiations in terms of social class, social stratification or lifestyles are generally ignored.

In some studies certain differential characteristics of whole cultures are contrasted. Sluzki (1979), for example, indicates how the egalitarian orientation of occidental cultures is in opposition with the autocratic values of Chinese and Latin culture. Sluzki, however, does not go on to integrate these factors into a framework which would allow a theory about the connections between culture and the family to be developed.

In terms of how it is defined, the meaning ascribed to the term 'culture' varies; it is sometimes referred to as a 'system of beliefs', and elsewhere as a 'system of rules' which govern behaviour (McGoldrick, 1982: p. 6).

In the UK concern with 'culture' within the mental health profession has been mainly manifested by professionals associated with the Transcultural Psychiatry Society in London. Although its membership is multidisciplinary, members primarily focus on ethnicity in the setting of the psychiatric hospital (e.g. Littlewood and Lipsedge, 1989; Rack 1982). Two papers on this theme (both within the context of family therapy) have been published in the UK (Lau, 1984; Hodes, 1985). While I am in agreement with the issues raised in both these papers, I specifically attempt here to define a conceptual framework which mediates between culture and family. This allows one to look at the ways in which culture organises cognitive and emotional elements within families. The context which interests me, therefore, is neither 'the culture', nor 'the family' alone; rather I attempt to construct a model to describe the connections between the two.

On both sides of the Atlantic, concern with 'culture' has thus developed as a consequence of dealing with 'ethnic' or 'immigrant' families. The concept of the family map, however, is important in the encounter between therapists and any family they deal with. The questions raised in attempts to understand families who come from 'other cultures' are also relevant to the achievement of a wider conceptual understanding of family processes and structures in general. This chapter addresses itself to the need to incorporate the concept of culture into the theoretical framework of family therapy.

Culture: structure and process

Anthropologists have for some time struggled with definitions of 'culture'. Arguably, anthropology is the attempt to define culture. Inherent in one of the most famous definitions provided by Tylor, is the problem, mentioned above, of perceiving culture as monolithic: 'that complex whole which includes knowledge, belief, art, morals, law, custom, and any other capabilities and habits acquired by man as a member of society' (Tylor, 1871). This definition does not explain the connection between culture and behaviour.

By explaining different types of behaviour within families as expressions of the rules of the (ethnic) groups with which these families identify themselves, many authors perceive behaviour as a mere actualisation of the structure. This is analogous to a musical performance merely representing the mechanical execution of the score. If culture and actual behaviour are thought to be automatically connected in this way, how can one account for the wide variation within cultures and, for that matter, for the processes and changes which occur within a specific culture (Bourdieu, 1977)? When dealing with 'ethnic' families in the American or British context, therapists are working with people who have already embarked upon a process of ethnic redefinition which entails the creation of new arrangements which do not necessarily 'fit' either those which predominate in their traditional settings or those of their new context.

Concepts are required which can aid the understanding of the relationship between the family and the wider culture and which can account for the 'movement' which occurs between the two. Geertz's (1973) concept of culture as a 'web of meaning' is important here because it leaves room for variations within the same culture. Another important contribution is that of Bateson (1958), who regards cultures as symbolic systems constructed by the scientist. Although family therapists differ in the way they intervene in families, there exists a consensus regarding the structural principle that patterns of interaction contain within themselves an image of the whole, i.e. they are expressions of the family organisation. The systemic approach, for example, argues that behaviour between members of the family expresses the rules of the system (Palazzoli *et al.*, 1980).

Two important ways of linking observable interaction and more abstract concepts have the following methodological implications which must be raised at this point:

(a) *The observed pattern is everything*
    It is my suggestion that teaching in family therapy has increasingly come to regard the idea of patterns of interaction as, literally, the entire reality which must be considered, rather than viewing them as an expression of something else, as a means of access to the family organisation. The danger implicit in this process is that of empiricism, of equating the family structure with the reality which can be directly observed. Those who believe that one can comprehend the world solely through the observation of patterns of interactions are the 'phenomenologists' (Bourdieu, 1972).

(b) *Patterns of interaction are merely a direct reflection of the structure*
    If patterns of interaction are regarded as expressions of something else, the assumption is that by observing the former one can derive the latter. In other words, the family structure may be arrived at through a collection of observations. However, one of the fundamental principles inherent in the notion of structure is that it does not refer to an empirically observable reality, but to models created from that reality. Lévi-Strauss (1958) has suggested that social relations are the raw material used in the construction of models that express the social structure. Structure lies not in the observable but in the constructed. Those who regard behaviour as the mere execution of the principles (whether these are termed organising principles, culture, or models) can be labelled as 'objectivists' (Bourdieu, 1972).

The objectivists emphasise the model whereas the phenomenologists believe that the 'truth' of the interaction lies in the interaction itself. The former rigidify behaviour and condemn the human being to imprisonment within the rules of the culture. People are regarded as mere performers who cannot, therefore, change. In contrast, the phenomenologists do not identify the matrix which gives meaning to processes (Bourdieu, 1972).

Conceptual framework

A number of concepts outlined below will be useful in establishing the connections between culture, family and patterns of behaviour.

(1) *The level of meaning of patterns of interaction.* One should consider the level of meaning as well as the behavioural and emotional characteristics of patterns of interaction. It is this level that reminds the observer that it is not possible, through observation alone, to understand that which is being observed. This is particularly obvious when one is dealing with the exotic. For instance, if a Briton goes to Africa and sees a man using a knife to scar an adolescent while a group of observers dance and sing, he might recognise the event as ritual, although its full meaning cannot be fully comprehended until it is placed in the context of the specific culture to which it belongs.

When dealing with the 'exotic' one is reminded that the rules of everyday life which are taken for granted are not, in fact, a 'given' part of the natural world, but are the product of a specific culture. In daily life these rules are so internalised that we are very rarely led to think about them. There exist, nevertheless, certain moments which force us to do this. Buñuel's film 'The Phantom of Liberty' vividly denaturalises the rules and thus makes the viewer more aware of the cultural origins of social rules. In an inspiring scene in this film, a family receives some guests who immediately sit around what we would perceive as a dining table. But instead of chairs, they sit on lavatories while making conversation, smoking, and reading newspapers. When a little girl complains that she is hungry, her mother reprimands her by reminding her that the subject should not be talked about at the table. One of the guests then excuses himself and retires to a small room at the end of the corridor – the equivalent of a toilet – and locks the door in order to eat in privacy. Thus, the film inverts patterns of everyday life in western societies so that eating is transformed into a private and polluted event whereas excreting becomes a social and public activity.

Every object in the above scene is familiar but the change of context creates the changed meaning. The perception of cultural arbitrariness is also facilitated when one's habitual way of thinking is disrupted. Crises are situations in which the rules which underlie family life can be thought about, possibly causing them to be changed or reinforced (Perelberg, 1980; 1980a).

(2) *The concepts of social structure and social organisation* (Firth, 1969), are useful mediators between the concept of culture on the one hand and that of patterns of interaction on the other. They stand respectively for form and process. Social organisation implies concrete activity which is arranged in sequences. Social structure is a conceptual, not an operational or descriptive tool. Both are functions of the culture. Here function is defined as that which establishes a relationship of interdependence (Bateson, 1958). The concept of culture lies at a higher level of abstraction than 'social structure' and 'social organisation' and neither of the latter two concepts can be derived from the former solely by deduction.

(3) *The family map*, another mediatory concept, lies at a lower level of abstraction. A map, I suggest, is the set of ideas which guide behaviour and emotions in everyday life, organise and systemise the world and transform its sensory dimensions into intelligible ones. Such a map establishes boundaries and shapes on otherwise undifferentiated territory. Family maps are a function of the culture, social structure and organisation but, once again, cannot be derived directly from these since maps involve a specific practice within the family. This implies the existence of specific configurations (shapes) within families. A family map may contain contradictory ideas and principles at different stages of the lifecycle; these may be held by the different members in the family. An example of these contradictory values can be seen in the case of a Hindu family who emigrated to England 16 years ago. The parents could still guide their lives according to the belief systems by which they had been brought up. The children, by contrast, are more in touch with the belief systems they had learned about at school. The family map would contain the conflicting ideas and expectations held by the two generations (see Spiegel, 1957). The concept of family map cuts across any notion of a dichotomy between the family and society as it emphasises both the specificity of the family and its articulation to the wider society.

It is possible to identify specific points of reference from which types of family maps can be traced. I will outline two models which lie at the two extremes of a continuum. I have designated these two types of family maps as hierarchical and symmetrical. The term 'symmetrical' was first used by Young and Willmott (1957) instead of 'egalitarian' to designate a 'new' type of family because of the marked differences that still exist between the genders. It should be noted, however, that the model of the symmetrical family presented in this paper uses a different set of reference points from those used by Young and Willmott since I am referring to both the organisational structure and webs of meaning within families. Hierarchical families are characterised by segregated activities and role relationships, while activities and relationships of symmetrical families are termed joint (Bott, 1957).

Family maps can be derived on the basis of the following points of reference:

(a)   The way in which activities within the home are organised along gender and generational lines.
(b)   The connections which partners maintain with their networks of friends and relatives (Bott, 1957).
(c)   Partners' attitudes to their children (Bernstein, 1974).
(d)   The way in which the family members perceive the connection between the individual and the world in which he or she is situated, i.e. whether they emphasise the autonomy of the individual (an egocentric model) or the role of the individual in relation to the family and the generations (the individual in a role, i.e. the person (Perelberg, 1980)), which is a sociocentric model. This will have implications both for the pattern of intimacy within the family (Bott, 1957; Firth, 1956), and for the perception family members have about the wider society (MacFarlane, 1978).

In terms of the relationship between gender roles, the hierarchical family is characterised by strict segregation of tasks. The woman is responsible for the bulk of the domestic work, which is strongly identified with femininity. The man will only do tasks, such as gardening or decorating, which are regarded as suitably male (Bott, 1957). The mother takes charge of most of the everyday care of the children, even though both parents are considered to be responsible for their socialisation and the inculcation of moral values. The father tends to be more distant towards his children and more frequently absent from the home. Even in symmetrical families where the father is generally more closely involved with the children, their intimacy tends to be confined to certain limited activities (Bott, 1957; Newson and Newson, 1963, 1970, 1976; and Lewis and O'Brien, 1987).

It is interesting to perceive how the ideology of 'what things should be like' contrasts with what actually happens in many families which aspire towards symmetry. Although in these symmetrical couples the fathers were in fact fairly closely involved in the educational and moral aspects of child rearing, all families complained of the difficulty of sharing equally the activities of child care (such as bathing, feeding, changing nappies) and stated that these remained predominantly the woman's sphere. This is in agreement with McKee's findings (1982), although she does not perceive this important difference between the ideal and the reality. Recent literature discussing fathers that do become closely involved with the upbringing of their children refer frequently to the 'lone father' (O'Brien, 1982; Hipgrave, 1982; Beckett, 1982; Russell, 1983). The activities of child care seem to be the last sphere that men share with women even in symmetrical families (see also research by Perelberg, 1983b).

In the symmetrical family, therefore, emphasis is placed on the sharing of household tasks and child rearing activities and the idea is one of equality in the conjugal partnership. Among these families, for example, greater stress is placed on the importance of women having independent careers. In the hierarchical family, great emphasis is placed on the positional relationship between members of the family: roles and moral rules are stressed and individuals refer constantly to their respective roles by, for example, stating 'you will do this because I say so and I am your father and you are my daughter'. In symmetrical families, the emphasis is on the autonomy and uniqueness of each individual (Bernstein, 1974). Hierarchical families are thus composed of persons defined in terms of their position or role in the system, whereas symmetrical families are composed of individuals (Perelberg, 1980; 1983a). In line with anthropological tradition I am here suggesting that different types of family structures are linked with different notions of the self and of its link with the family and the wider society.

These two types of families are also associated with two types of network (Bott, 1957). A family's network is that set of people with whom the family maintains relationships. The members of the network may or may not know each other and do not necessarily meet independently. In the hierarchical family the segregation of roles within the home is reflected in the segregation of the relationships outside it. Thus, the husband has his own friends and the wife has hers, although her network more usually seems to comprise kin rather than friends (Young and Willmott, 1952). In symmetrical families, husbands and wives tend to have more common friends (Bott, 1957; Perelberg, 1983b).

It should be stressed that the concepts of segregated and joint conjugal role relationships are quite distinct from Minuchin's concept of disengaged and enmeshed families (Minuchin *et al*, 1978). Firstly, Minuchin was characterising types of pathologies within families and indicated specific guidelines about how these families' patterns should be changed. If, on the one hand, he claimed that a certain level of enmeshment and disengagement was present in any family, he also stressed, on the other hand, that either of the extremes of enmeshment and disengagement indicate areas of possible pathology. This is not true of joint and segregated role relationships which, being sociological categories, present predominant patterns of social organisation. Secondly, Minuchin was identifying transactional styles within families rather than social roles, as is the concern here. I would suspect, however, that enmeshed families would predominantly have joint role-relationships and loose-knit networks although, of course, not all families with loose-knit networks and joint role-relationships can be described as enmeshed.

These two models, hierarchical and symmetrical (see Table 8.1), do not deny the empirical diversity of family forms, but are constructs which suggest that several variables must be considered in the attempt to identify specific patterns of family organisations and family maps (Bernstein, 1974; Edgell, 1980; Perelberg, 1983b; Rapport *et al.*, 1982; 1982a). The establishment of such structural principles for identifying family maps cannot be equated with descriptive categories such as nuclear, one-parent or extended families. These merely describe phenomena rather than establish their organising principles. A one-parent family, for example, could be either hierarchical or symmetrical depending on the points of reference which constitute its map.

Table 8.1   Types of family maps

	Hierarchical	Symmetrical
Unit of analysis	The person (roles): sociocentric model. The biological individual is more clearly embedded in a network of social relationships.	The autonomous individual: egocentric model
Role-relationship	Segregated	Joint
Perception of children	Roles stressed	Individual qualities stressed
Network	Close-knit	Loose-knit

At this point, it is possible to draw the conceptual framework which establishes the links between the various levels of analysis: culture, social structure, social organisation, family maps (ranging from hierarchical to symmetrical), and patterns of interaction (which must include the level of meaning because it most clearly refers back to the existence of family maps).

A hierarchical relationship exists between these various levels. Thus, if one moves from the patterns of interaction towards the concept of culture, one is moving towards a higher level of abstraction. Each level is a function of all the others in that there exists a relationship of interdependence, but none can be derived deductively from knowledge of any of the others, as there is always a new dimension to be added. Greater attention must be paid to the diversity of specific processes and events when one moves towards patterns of interaction and, conversely, moving towards the concepts of culture involves the integration of additional analytical concepts (Fig. 8.1).

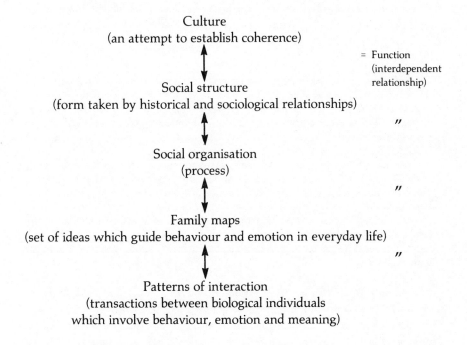

Fig. 8.1   Conceptual framework establishing links between the various levels of analysis.

I will now indicate the way in which these issues are relevant to clinical practice by discussing four families who came to the Department for Children and Adolescents at the Maudsley Hospital and the Marlborough Family Service in London. All the names and identifying details about the families have been changed in order to protect their privacy and confidentiality. Both units are part of the NHS and serve a population derived from a diversity of ethnic origins and social classes. The examples illustrate the usefulness of the concept of the family map when creating a therapeutic alliance in family therapy (Gurman, 1982). The first, second and fourth families are hierarchical; the third is a symmetrical family. The first two (who were seen by colleagues at the Maudsley Hospital) are examples of first interviews with families where doubt existed as to whether one was dealing with a 'cultural pattern' – derived from a 'different culture' in the first case, or from a 'different class' in the second – or with a pathological system. The third family is an example of an idiosyncratic pattern of organisation which might have provoked the therapist to take a moralistic stance. The fourth family will be discussed in greater detail as it affords an example in which the family map was taken carefully into account.

Case study 1

The unit which came to the clinic was composed of the parents, the Bertorellis, their five children and one grandchild. The parents were both in their fifties, and had emigrated from Italy to England some 25 years ago. Of the five children, Rosana, 24 years old, was married and living in her own home; Sonia, 22 years old, was also married and living in her own home; Carla, 19 years old, Roberto, 16 years old, and Mariana, 14, lived at home.

Carla had attempted suicide and was referred to the Maudsley by the emergency clinic. During the first interview it became clear that the father mediated between the family and the outside world. He translated into Italian for his wife although she both understood what was being said and could make herself understood in English. Their conjugal role-relationship can be described as segregated. During the session the therapist elicited from Carla the information that she had tried to kill herself because she could not stand her parents' pressure about what she was going to do with her life.

She wanted to be able to leave home and have a life 'of her own', but she said her father could not understand her desire. According to the father, Carla had everything she wanted at home and the outside world was a dangerous place. Even worse, in his eyes, Carla's leaving home would mean that the family would lose its honour. He kept repeating that he was her father and he knew what was best. Family roles were emphasised: Carla was not an autonomous individual but a person. In their view, Carla would cease to exist for the family if she left home. The therapist was able to discover from the father that although he would suffer deeply if Carla died, the possibility of her leaving home presented an even worse threat as his worries about the dangers she would face would be unbearable and the family's honour would be at stake.

After the session, the therapist reported that he felt that although he had understood what had been happening, he had not been able to make his message heard. After discussing his interventions, it became clear that he had treated family members as if they were all equal and had stressed that they were all intelligent individuals who had expressed different opinions. I pointed out that this was a hierarchical family in which the positional relationships between the members were crucial. The same message phrased in those terms and taking into consideration the family's map would more easily be heard and understood by the family.

The family therapist in this case is not dealing with a 'cultural' problem, but with a family which has a specific history and which is negotiating contradictions within its map. There are conflicting values at stake: the parents and older siblings emphasise the values which comprise a hierarchical configuration (segregation of roles, positional roles, emphasis on the person) and the middle daughter attempts to include the notion of herself as an autonomous individual. Spiegal (1957) has suggested that amongst minority families some conflicts can be understood in terms of discrepancies in culture value orientations between social roles. An awareness of the family map in this case was vital for the formulation of successful interventions.

Case study 2

The Fisher family was typical of traditional English working-class families (see Bernstein, 1974; Firth, 1969; Rapoport *et al.*, 1982; Young and Willmott, 1957). It was composed of Mr and Mrs Fisher, both of whom were in their late fifties; their youngest daughter Joanna, who was 16 years old; Lynn, who was 31 years old, divorced and lived in her parents' home with her seven-year-old daughter; and Susan, married with two children, who lived nearby. The family had been referred because of Joanna's refusal to go to school, her fearfulness, and her lack of friends.

The distribution of roles within the family became clear during the very first session. Father was the gate keeper, the mediator between the public and the domestic domain; the mother was in charge of the latter, the care of the house and the children. The father was the first to answer the therapist's question about what the problem was, giving his wife permission to speak. He also stressed that this was a 'mother's matter', since it concerned their daughter. In the following segments the therapist is violating the pathways of communication utilised by the family by insisting that the father speaks to his daughter directly.

1st segment:
MR F: 'The wife better begin because she knows better than I do . . . . She knows more about it, obviously.'
THERAPIST: 'Obviously?'
MR F: 'Yes, because my daughter would consult with my wife more than she would do with me, because I'm not there all day, am I?'

2nd segment:
The therapist asks how mother and father deal with Joanna's problem.
MR F: 'If Joanna has a problem and she comes to me, I try to solve it.'

THERAPIST: 'I wonder if what you said got through to Joanna.'
MR F: 'I said that if she has any problem she can come to me.'
THERAPIST: 'I wonder if it got through to her.'
MR F: 'I don't get your drift. That's why I'm talking to you.'
THERAPIST: 'I don't know whether Joanna heard what you said because you're talking to me.'
MR F: 'Of course she heard.'
THERAPIST: 'Has she taken your drift?'
MR F: 'Of course she has. She knows that if she has any problem she can come to me, but prefers to go to her mother.'

The Fishers represent another example of a hierarchical family in which there exists a strict segregation of roles according to which the mother is responsible for the domestic domain. The therapist is violating the family's rules by insisting that the father speaks to his daughter, bypassing her mother. In an apparently familiar pattern – that of an English family – the therapist did not perceive the 'exotic' element, i.e. the unfamiliar rules which, in this case, concerned the segregation of tasks in the domestic domain.

The third segment indicates the boundaries of the family, which is not the household of people who live together (Laslett, 1972), but parents, children and grandchildren. The matrifocal emphasis is thus revealed.

3rd segment:
MRS F: 'There are three daughters. One of them lives with me, the other lives near me because I need to babysit for my grand-daughter when she goes out. Actually she seems more part of the family as compared to a separate unit because we see her daily.'
THERAPIST: 'How old is your daughter?'
MRS F: 'Nearly 31.'
THERAPIST: 'And she seems part of the family too, is that right Mrs Fisher?'
MRS F: 'Of course. She is one of my daughters, so she is part of my family, even if she lived 100 miles away.'
THERAPIST: 'This is a very close family that cares very much for its members . . . . This is not unusual, but it is not necessarily obvious to me. Some families are not that close and don't worry so much about their members.'
MR F: 'I don't agree with you. When you have children, they are part of the family and they are part of the family for the rest of their lives . . . . Normally, a family keeps together.'
THERAPIST: 'Do you agree with that, Mrs Fisher?'
MRS F: 'As a family unit we are very close, my daughters phone, if I don't see them . . . . She comes down when she can. As I say, it's a unit . . . .'

The fourth segment stresses the opposition between the home and the outside world, the family and strangers, 'I and them' which has been widely discussed in the literature on the English traditional working class (Bernstein, 1974; Hoggart, 1957). It also expresses the positional role of the father in relation to his daughter as he tells her the principles of reality. At the end of the segment the father's perception of Joanna's problem is also revealed, not as an individual problem but as a stage in her lifecycle, the same one that her sister Susan had gone through when she was Joanna's age. It is once more the position of the person that is emphasised.

4th segment:

MR F: 'Home is a refuge. Any problems you have outside you can leave outside, because home is a refuge. . . . So whatever happens outside, you always have got, how I can describe it? It's a refuge, home is a refuge. Home is to be enjoyed.'

THERAPIST: 'What do you tell Mrs Fisher about this?'

MR F: 'I don't have to tell my wife anything. We have lived together for so long that our minds are the same . . . . After you've lived together for so long you don't have to communicate every little thing to one another, right?'

MRS F: 'That's right.'

THERAPIST: 'You don't have to communicate?'

MRS F: 'Oh, we do talk.'

MR F: 'We do talk, but it's not necessary.'

THERAPIST: 'Can I leave you with something to work on while I talk to my colleagues? Can I ask you to outline to Mr Fisher the kinds of things that perhaps are not so easy to convey by instinct, something that maybe you're aware of that your husband should know but finds it difficult to sometimes.'

MR F: 'But you still don't know what the problem is. You seem to be more concerned with the wife and I.'

THERAPIST: 'I suppose my first instinct when I meet a family . . . is not to move too fast.'

MR F: 'I supposed you'd go straight to the point and find out what the problem is . . . we haven't touched it yet. . . I know what you want to find out, what sort of parents we are, and I appreciate that. The problem with Jo is adolescence, from a child to an adult, a given period, say from 12 to 17 when they're school children and they turn into adults. It was the same with my other daughter . . . .'

Again in this segment the therapist did not pay sufficient attention to the rules about family life that the family was expressing: Mrs Fisher's expertise in matters relating to her daughter and Mr Fisher's role as the family spokesman and intermediary with the outside world. This suggests that an exercise of fundamental importance for a family therapist is to try and find out (and understand) the 'exotic' in families he (the therapist) considers to be 'familiar'.

Case study 3

The Donalds were referred because of Debbie's continuing refusal to attend school, her unhappiness and lack of friends, and the recurrent abdominal pains which she experienced. I saw this family for a total of 15 sessions over a period of more than a year. Debbie came to the first session in tears, with her parents. It became clear during the interviews that the composition of the family was complex. Although they lived in the same house with their three children – Sylvia (20 years old), Robert (18 years old) and Debbie (13 years old) – Mr and Mrs Donald (who were 72 and 42 years old respectively) no longer slept together; they had 'separated'. They shared the same house with Mrs Donald's new partner, Mr O'Hara (22 years old) and their three children, Gemma (5 years old), Jo (4 years old), and Sarah (2 years old). All of them were invited to attend subsequent interviews.

The Donalds presented their family map as that of a 'democratic', undifferentiated unit in which everyone had an equal right to express their point of view. The fact that the criterion of age, for example, was not important in terms of ranking, was indicated by the ages of Mr Donald, Mrs Donald and Mr O'Hara. In the first session, as they reluctantly told me about the composition of their household, Mr and Mrs Donald were also testing my reaction. When my response was simply to invite everybody to come to the next session in order to help Debbie more effectively, they immediately saw that I was not taking a moralistic stance. Nevertheless, they were clearly on their guard at the next session.

At this stage the fact that I was both an anthropologist and a foreigner was of immense help. Because I was a foreigner they could assume that I did not know how uncommon their household arrangement might be, and as an anthropologist I had been trained to be aware of the diversity of lifestyles. I therefore accepted their decision to be a three-parent family living in the same household and recognised their family map in which both the autonomy of each individual and joint activities were emphasised.

Gradually, I reached a basic agreement with the family. At that specific moment in time something was making Debbie unhappy. The family would have to help me find out what it was, and in order to do so latent rules of family life would have to be clarified even though, in normal everyday life, the rules need not be articulated. I also said, at that stage, that all societies had at least two principles of differentiation, sex and age (see La Fontaine, 1978). The latter in particular seemed to me to be rather ambiguous in their family. The strategic component of the therapeutic contract with the family was that while I respected the idiosyncratic, loose three-parent family organisation which was consciously chosen by the family, I also reached an agreement about the notions of gender, hierarchy and boundaries between the generations.

Throughout the therapy a tension was maintained between the notions of the family as a democratic unit and those of boundaries and hierarchies. My hypothesis was that as Sylvia was about to leave home, Debbie was placed in an ambiguous position. She was, on the one hand, Mr and Mrs Donald's daughter, i.e. one of the children in the household. On the other hand, the existence of Mr and Mrs Donald as a parental couple implied that either Mr O'Hara was one of the children, or that he was available as a possible partner for Debbie. This ambiguity was increased by Mrs Donald's feelings of incompetence in looking after the home and the three smaller children and her constant requests for help from Debbie. By not going to school, Debbie was staying in the house and taking over from her mother. She also helped to maintain the balance between the two families. While she was at home, Mr Donald still retained a role since they had all decided, in the past, that it was better to live together for the sake of the children.

Potentially, they all had something to lose if Debbie were to get better and grow up. The crucial aspect of the therapeutic process, therefore, implied the acceptance of the three-parent family structure within the same household, at the same time as boundaries were traced between parents and children, mother and daughter, around all the siblings, and then around older and younger siblings.

Case study 4

The Suma family comprised the mother and father and nine children (five girls and four boys aged between 32 and 16 years). My first contact with them was through a telephone call from their eldest, 32-year-old daughter, Simena, saying that her 24-year-old brother Sunjay had become mute and refused to get up in the morning. She asked for an appointment which the parents and seven of the nine children attended.

The Sumas were Hindus, East African–Asians, who had come to England for political reasons, having had to flee their home country leaving all their property and money behind. When they arrived in this country they were helped by Mrs Suma's brother to open a business. Mr Suma started to drink heavily. The four eldest sisters took charge of the business and the older brother went to college. The father, therefore, had completely lost his position as the family's provider. There had been conflicts between husband and wife who decided not to speak to each other again. They had not spoken to each other for some 12 years before they came to the session and to have changed this situation would have involved a 'loss of face' for each of them.

In the two preceding years the following events took place in rapid succession. The third sister got married and emigrated to America. The fourth sister left the family business to marry a Muslim. The father had been very upset by this and also stopped speaking to her. She was also on non-speaking terms with the two sisters still involved in the business. The 31-year-old daughter was about to get married which would then leave Simena, the eldest, to look after the 'family business' on her own. The business, a newsagent's shop, was located on the other side of London. She lived there on her own and at the weekends went back to the family home. Two years previously Sunjay had become involved with a Muslim 'guru' who had converted him to Islam. He had been told by his parents to go and live with Simena because they thought that by looking after the family business he might 'become himself again'.

During the first session, two versions of Sunjay's problems were put forward. The father definitely thought Sunjay should see a psychiatrist as he had become 'kinky like' after his contact with the guru. According to the second version, there was a communication problem within the family and Sunjay, because he was so sensitive, was more vulnerable than the others. The three older children particularly supported this view and wanted to employ me to get the parents to talk to each other.

My hypothesis at this stage was derived from looking at the family map. This was a hierarchical family with segregated role-relationships where, due to historical circumstances and their specific life history, the relationships between the genders and the generations had become inverted. The women had taken over the task of providing for the family and the children that of looking after their parents. At that specific moment in the lifecycle Simena, after her sisters had left the family business, was at risk of remaining, for ever, the only one responsible for looking after the business, her parents, and Sunjay.

Silence had been used by the family to deal with major contradictions. These included the inversion of positions between the sexes and the generations. The mother and the father had stopped speaking to each other after coming to England and the fourth daughter was not speaking to the family because of her marriage to a Muslim. By becoming silent in his own sister's house, Sunjay was attempting to activate the most powerful person in the family, who also had most to lose at that point in time, to try to do something about the situation. Simena had in fact persistently tried to talk to each parent about Sunjay's problem but because they could not talk to each other, she became a prisoner of her role as mediator. By the end of the first session, I realised that to agree that there was a 'communication problem' in the family would only further alienate Mr Suma. I decided to support his position and asked a psychiatrist to see Sunjay.

His diagnosis was that there was nothing psychiatrically wrong with Sunjay and this gave added impetus to our meetings. I accepted the father's idea that the guru had made Sunjay 'kinky' and proceeded to ask the family to discuss with Sunjay whether he was at that point Hindu or Muslim. It turned out that none was sure of the answer. I labelled Sunjay's silence as an expression of the fact that he did not know who he was. I asked whether they knew of any ceremony which would allow a Muslim to become a Hindu again, in case Sunjay wanted to go through it, and Mr Suma turned out to be the only person in the family who was knowledgeable about religious matters. During the following session, Sunjay discussed with his father his possible re-conversion to Hinduism. The conversations went on for weeks and then Mr Suma organised a ceremony, which Sunjay underwent, a few months later. Throughout the process the therapist did not request that the mother and the father should talk to each other directly. The men in the family had their role re-instated and this allowed Simena greater flexibility and freedom from her previously rigid position.

The therapeutic interventions employed here required careful tracking of the family map. While this included the observation of patterns of interaction in the room (the mother and the father not speaking to each other, Simena acting as mediator between the two, father being largely ignored in the first session, etc.), what these meant to the family also had to be considered. The interventions which followed were then syntonic with the principles of the family map.

It is clear that the concept of culture would not have been sufficient to understand what was happening within this family. There was a dynamic process taking place in which roles and rules were being re-defined and re-negotiated. These new arrangements did not necessarily 'fit' either those predominant in their traditional context nor those of the new setting. The concept of family map allows for the dynamics of the process to be considered.

Conclusion

This chapter has introduced the term family map as a concept that can be employed to mediate between the family and the culture to which it belongs. Although maps are always present in the encounters between therapists and their families, it is only when faced with 'exotic' families that the therapist becomes aware of their existence. This chapter suggests that this concept should be brought to the centre of the conceptual framework in family therapy.

I have suggested a conceptual framework for the analysis of the links between family and culture by defining and indicating the connections between the concepts of culture, social structure, social organisation, hierarchical and symmetrical types of family maps, and patterns of interaction. In proposing this framework, the pitfalls of both phenomenologists (who believe that patterns of interaction represent all the reality which needs to be considered) and objectivists (who perceive patterns of interaction as a mere execution of the structure) have been pointed out. The proposed conceptual framework indicates a hierarchical relationship of successively higher levels of abstraction leading from 'patterns of interaction' towards the concept of 'culture'. Each level is a function of all the others (and all are interdependent) but none can be derived deductively from knowledge of any of the others as there always exists a new dimension which must be added.

We then looked at the clinical implications and applications of this framework. Of the four families which were presented, three were characterised as having a predominantly hierarchical map, and one a symmetrical map. Some of the pitfalls faced by the therapists dealing with the four families were indicated. Although the therapist treating the first family (an immigrant family) was aware of his unfamiliarity with their cultural background, he did not build up the family map in terms of the points of reference I have suggested. Thus he conveyed his initial message as if he was dealing with autonomous individuals rather than persons invested in roles.

In the second case, the therapist was unaware of this unfamiliarity as he was dealing with an English and therefore an apparently familiar family map. Differences between himself and the family were regarded by the therapist as indicating pathology. These families presented, in fact, examples of family maps involving segregated role relationships. It is clear that many other families in which the same patterns exist cannot be described as pathological. The third family was an idiosyncratic symmetrical family in which, by respecting the arrangement consciously adopted by the family, I was able to establish a strategic framework which made it possible to explore their vulnerable areas. In the fourth, the hierarchical family, the interventions were congruent with the understanding of the family map.

The analysis of the encounter between therapist and family in the four cases leads me to suggest that the distance between the therapist's own map and the family's should be identified at the beginning of the therapeutic process. This awareness should influence the therapeutic model chosen by the therapist. A strategic model, one that focuses on the literal meaning of messages transmitted by families whose maps differ greatly from the therapist's, is more likely to succeed in engaging such families than challenges which ignore the elements of those families' maps. The therapist should, thus, be able to identify the following at the outset:

- The main views held by the family about the genders and the generation.
- The way the main activities in the house are organised in terms of gender differentiation.
- What connections are maintained with the networks of friends and relatives.
- How the children are perceived by adults in the family.

- Whether there exists an emphasis on the autonomy of the individual in the family (an egocentric model) or on the role of the individual in relation to the family (a sociocentric model).
- The way in which these arrangements are expressed in the observable patterns of interaction within the family.

In the literature it has been suggested that a strategic model of therapy should be used depending on the stage of the therapeutic process (Stanton, 1981), or the type of pathology exhibited by the family (Madanes, 1982). In a 'cartography' of the research literature in the field, Gurman and Kniskern (1982) have suggested that three major sources of variables are likely to influence the results of family therapy, namely other treatment factors, patient factors and family factors. I am suggesting here that an aspect which needs to be considered when joining with a family is the therapist's familiarity with the map of the family with which he or she is dealing.

This chapter has pointed out the risk faced by family therapists of 'colonising' families that seek treatment when they attempt to reconstruct family patterns without concerning themselves with the meaning which those families attribute to their own lifestyles. The diversity of social contexts becomes reduced to pathological structures. If families exist only in culture, meaning can only be attributed through language, and the understanding of a specific pattern cannot be achieved through observation or logical inference alone. It thus becomes necessary to ask the individual members of the family about their own perception of what they are doing so that their meanings can be taken into consideration. What family members say and do, and even their unconscious structures, are in the final analysis derived from, and only exist within, the symbolic systems at their disposal.

Note

Dumont (1966) has distinguished between the biological individual, present in all cultures, and the 'individual as a rational being'. This latter concept has a very recent history, having been developed in the 17th and 18th centuries in occidental civilisation. Dumont argues that in traditional societies the minimal unit of social life is the collective man, i.e. 'the stress is placed on the society as a whole' (1966: p. 44) whereas in modern societies this unit is the elementary man. Dumont's reasoning is developed only on a diachronic level whereas I have suggested the co-existence of different emphases, on the person and on the individual, in different types of family structures, within the same society.

Acknowledgements

This chapter is based on presentations to the 4th International Conference in Family Therapy in Tel Aviv in 1983, to the National Conference of the Association for Family Therapy in York, 1983, and on later seminars and workshops presented for the Diploma in Family Therapy at the Institute of Psychiatry and University College London, and to the Institute of Family Therapy, London. I am especially grateful to Dr Alan Cooklin, Dr Christopher Dare and Ms Ann Miller for inspiring discussions. The cases were taken from the clinics at the Department for Children and Adolescents at the Maudsley Hospital and the Marlborough Family Service, London.

Chapter 9

Racism and Psychotherapy; Working With Racism in the Consulting Room: An Analytical View

LENNOX THOMAS

Racism can exist in many forms in our society and can affect our lives in many ways. Ideas of white superiority and white supremacy form part of the fabric of UK (and other) societies and play a part in the way that white people relate to non-white people. The question I would like to pose here is: what makes the dealings in a consulting room between a white therapist and a black patient 'different'? What are the processes which the therapist needs to go through in order to disentangle themselves from the structural racism of the society in which they live and where they were raised?

The working through of issues of racism seems to be relatively unimportant for the training analysis of candidates. It has proved difficult for analytical societies to deal with this issue, perhaps because training analysts and supervisors alike have little awareness of the significance of race and racism in the therapeutic process. These professionals have not hitherto viewed themselves as needing to address the issue, since most psychotherapy is conducted as a private, fee-paying activity. Given this 'social' location of psychotherapy and psychoanalysis, the issue is never opened to public debate: the implication is that an individual pays for a service and is free to choose to leave, or to remain, depending on the way that they view the quality of the service.

This view assumes an individual rational choice on the part of the patient: however, therapists employed by the National Health Service, or other agencies, must follow the policies of the organisation in question and might therefore be expected to address this issue. It seems likely, however, that white workers in this field are not yet fully aware of the existence of or motivation for their own or others' racist attitudes and assumptions. The quest for 'awareness' has always been one of the aims of psychoanalytic therapies, and awareness of the part that structural and personal racism plays in clinical work should not be an exception. Self-awareness and self-knowledge also constitute therapeutic tools and a resistance to explore this issue renders the therapist incapable of helping either black or white patients who need to explore this material.

Sexism, like racism, is an issue for psychotherapy. The Women's Therapy Centre in North London provides both clinical and theoretical information on its therapeutic procedures with women patients (Laurence, 1987; Ernst and McGuire, 1987). It remains to be seen if wider training institutes can incorporate this data into their own therapeutic methods. Racism, even if it is neither violent nor overt, is harmful to black people, just as sexism is harmful to women. Subtle racism attaches to a system of assumptions and negative stereotypes about black people that is countertherapeutic. Racism, wherever it arises, denies the black person individual characteristics – seen as normal or ordinary – which white people are held to possess. Characteristics are ascribed to black people which may be based on centuries of distortion. These beliefs lie within all of us and are certainly evoked in the powerful setting of the therapeutic encounter.

Thus, the black individual in therapy risks being viewed simply as a representative type, constituted in turn from stereotypes. The white therapist, on the other hand, as a member of a society which has its own pervasive, negative views about black people, will have difficulty in separating out the black individual from his or her race (Curry, 1964). It is extremely difficult for any form of racism, accrued from a lifetime of socialisation, to be brought to personal awareness, yet this is indeed what needs to take place, so that our practice is not dominated by what can be termed 'societal racism'. In order to work effectively across cultures and with people of different colour, psychotherapists, I would suggest, need first to attend to their own racism, their own prejudices, and their own projections on other racial and cultural groups. Personal attitudes and assumptions need to be re-worked and re-examined. In order to lend emphasis to this, this chapter might have been given the subtitle 'the therapist prepares'.

The therapist's part in the encounter

The psychotherapist, like the client, brings to the therapeutic situation fears and problems transferred from the past (Salzberger–Wiltenberg, 1970). The therapist will have had the opportunity to deal with these in a training analysis. If the training analyst is black and the candidate white, then there might seem to be an opportunity here for this to be considered; however, there might also be a need in this situation to deny any differences in order to preserve the therapy as a 'safe place'. When this happens a valuable opportunity is missed. Then again, the possibility of a white candidate and a white therapist engaging with this material would be remote: this, however, is the usual situation in psychotherapy training.

It is clear from other writers in the field that both race and gender play an important part in therapeutic interaction: 'the process of gender as a functioning reality within the psychoanalytic situation makes it clear that other realities, such as ethnic background, social position, and language must influence the emotions, interactions and level of understanding of both analyst and patient' (Allport, 1986). Indeed, *not* acknowledging the gender or colour of one's patient can be seen as a form of pathology since this serves to deny certain processes. In the case of colour, white therapists often report that 'they do not notice' that their patients are black, and indeed 'treat all patients the same'. Given the power that the professional has for the establishment of reality in the relationship, there is an urgent need for white therapists to recognise the pathological aspects that might, albeit unknowingly, be employed in their dealings with their own racism as well as what might be brought by their patients. The systemic effect of 'racism' is little understood in our society and likewise in psychotherapy. Many workers find themselves denying any part of this system, neither recognising nor diagnosing its action or its after-effects.

The actual practice of racism is too often equated simply with the activities and beliefs of extreme right wing organisations. Racism, however, is not just a hatred of, or a conscious belief in the inferiority of, black people. Nor is it just physical violence. Disavowal of a person's 'different' existence is in itself a way of not recognising the degree to which this pervasive system operates in groups and in the individual. Inevitably, racism has a detrimental effect on social and personal relationships. Not only is this evident in relationships between black and white people but between black people themselves.

As an illustration of this point, a child psychotherapist, a white woman, working in a culturally and racially mixed area, reported to me that she could not give black children black dolls for the purpose of playwork. She was adamant that her own personal upbringing had taught her to treat people with respect regardless of their colour or background. She was surprised, when reflecting on the matter, that her reluctance to use black dolls with black children was a wish to protect them; she did not want them to have something inferior. This was what the black dolls represented to her. White is considered standard and normal, and black special, abnormal or inferior.

One is left to speculate on the unspoken meanings that are conveyed to and internalised by black children who grow up in a society where both black and white people are denied access to an important part of their world – the valid representation and experience of their blackness. This can only be countertherapeutic: the symbols represented through white dolls can provoke only a limited response since white and whiteness is only part of a child's world. It would be a most unusual situation for white children in therapy to be given only black dolls by a therapist.

The particular therapist cited above later felt that her training and experience were called into question, and she was genuinely confused: why had such an issue never been raised in her clinic before? She wondered why she had not been given the opportunity to explore the symbols attached to the black dolls since they were important working tools. She understood that it was her protective feelings towards her black child patients that made her want to shelter them from the fact of their own blackness whilst they were in her room. She did not fully realise that she was also protecting herself from her whiteness, and the children's realisation of this difference between them in therapy.

It is because some therapists may believe, at levels sometimes not available to them, that black people are inferior, that they protect themselves and their patients from dealing with issues of blackness and whiteness. In so doing they also 'protect' themselves from the real social experiences which are encountered by black patients as a consequence of being black. Psychotherapy is a 'social institution' and therefore will reflect what takes place in society. As a therapeutic endeavour, however, directed at change and given the appropriate training and conditions, there is an opportunity for transcending and understanding these constraints.

The white therapist and the black patient

Being white or being black affects the development of people in society no less than being male or female. Discrimination and racism play a part not only in our material lives, but also in our mental lives. Our psychological development will be in some way shaped by our experiences and by how we see ourselves and how others see us. A white person raised in the confidence of the 'superiority' of their whiteness might possess knowledge of this superiority at various levels. A therapeutic encounter with a black patient could provide a certain fit, in which the black patient 'knew their place', a knowledge reflected in other relationships with white people. Put, oversimplistically, in a society where people in positions of power and authority are white, the scene could be set for a simple re-enactment of other social scenarios. It is the therapist's task to recognise and explore pathological fit along racial lines in the transference. This, of course, is not easy when the countertransference is also powerfully bent on enactment.

Andrew Curry, in his paper, 'Myths, transference and the black psychotherapist', puts forward the concept of the 'pre-transference'. This he describes as the ideas, fantasies, and values ascribed to the black psychotherapist and his race which are held by the white patient long before the two meet for the first time in the consulting room. Brought up in the society which holds negative views about black people, the white patient will have to work through this before engaging properly in the transference. The white psychotherapist too will need to deal with this when working with black patients. As I mentioned earlier, this is not the same thing as the personal countertransference which should be dealt with in the training analysis. This pre-transference is constituted of material from the past: fairy tales, images, myths and jokes. Current material, in the form of media images, may serve to top up this unconscious store of negative attributes.

As has been said, little attention is paid to racism in psychotherapy training and practice. To a large extent, the solution to these difficulties lies within the existing psychoanalytic method itself. Dealing with splitting, projection, defences, symbols, and the exploration of the unconscious is the accepted model for analytic work as it is for engaging with issues of race in the consulting room. Racism (intentional or otherwise) is a functional part of the ego structure and we each need to know what it acts in the service of. The practising therapist or analyst can often find themselves derailed by these issues with the emergence of their own countertransference through conventional attitudes to their patients' race. The following examples are offered to illustrate this:

Example 1

A young black woman on her way to analysis was spat on by an elderly white woman in a bus queue. She arrived tearful and distressed. On telling her analyst that she had called the woman, 'a wicked old cow', the analyst's first response was that she should not have reacted in this way because the woman was quite old. The analyst considered that to ignore the matter would have been the best way of dealing with it. The patient responded by feeling angry but could not express this until several sessions later. She felt that her analyst was not concerned about her feelings, but was protective to another white person whom the analyst did not even know. The patient felt that her analyst (someone who had been her analyst over the previous two years) still did not have any real concern for, or understanding of, her situation. Her subsequent departure from therapy was caused by what seemed to her the analyst's unworked feelings about race which remained an immovable object between them. The treatment came to an abrupt end, the patient angry and bitter about the trust she had invested in the relationship. I learned that the

racial difference between the patient and analyst had never been acknowledged before this incident.

Example 2

A white psychotherapist brought a case for supervision: a young black patient
with whom she had been working for several months. They appear to have
a good working relationship. She reports that he is diligent and makes good
use of his treatment. As a child he had suffered at the hands of a tyrannical
mother who totally dominated him and still attempts to do so. He recognises
the pain and fear he has suffered as a child and is making an attempt to
renegotiate his relationship with his mother. He has, however, a strong need
to gloss over the past and to preserve his mother from his wish to retaliate
and attack. His current dilemma in therapy is that, after having found work
after a long period of unemployment, he seems unhappy and unsettled. He
works for a company where his immediate supervisor is overtly racially
abusive. He feels that this man is always finding fault with him as a person
and with the work that he performs. In therapy he expresses this pain openly
and uses his sessions to talk about it. At times he rages in anger whilst at
others he is low and desolate. His therapist reports that she feels paralysed
and totally useless, not knowing how she can help him. She feels that his
problems are real, external, and that there is nothing that she can do in
therapy. Indeed, *she* was low and desolate.

Here, it is difficult for the therapist to recognise that the unconscious does
not distinguish between colour as far as the perpetrators of pain are
concerned, and that in this case it was some of the pain suffered at the hands
of his mother that was now resurrected. This connection did cross her mind
but she feared using it as a bridge for an interpretation: her patient's dilemma
at work, she considered, must be a separate matter. She could not see that, for
her, it was a separate matter, while for the patient, still the child in pain, there
was not such a distinction, only repetition. Of course, making the link was not
going to be easy but it had to be made. My concern was, that if the bringing
together was not made soon, the young man might be pushed into acting out
the original conflict and that his violence against his supervisor might be
boundless. Of course, to him there would be rational conscious reasons, but
it might also be his downfall. The problem, with its genesis in his childhood,
and now bound up with his outer and inner world, could become a matter for
litigation. The therapist, however, feared that her patient would reject any
attempt to link the present with the past. It seemed that she needed to
understand that denial and rejection are the stuff of which psychotherapy is
made. The unconscious never readily yields up its peculiar fruit unless it is re-
enacted (or acted out). A paper by Mary Twyman (1984) notes that acting out

may take the form of aggressive behaviour directed at the self or at others. She adds that, whether it occurs in the session or not, it must be understood in relation to the transference, since, classically, it is a basic refusal to recognise that transference. I wondered whether or not this therapist had difficulty in recognising her countertransference here. Her own anger at her patient's persecuting supervisor was giving way to her passive participation in an attack on him. She was outraged by his overt racism and somehow this itself was clouding the treatment. She herself was on the point of acting, with or alongside, her patient. To an extent, she was of course right in saying that there was a real problem for her patient in coping with racist abuse at work, but first she had to address for herself the issues and feelings raised about racism and how this affected her practice.

The black therapist and the white patient

In general, there is little material on this situation and its absence perhaps reflects the fact that few black mental health professionals have undergone additional training in psychoanalysis or psychotherapy. Thus the profession is almost totally white, with few exceptions. It is not surprising, therefore, that a black psychotherapist when initially seeing a white patient is sometimes met with surprise. The relationship in the consulting room presents the patient with a conundrum. The situation of the black person as 'an expert' goes against conventional information received about black people. The patient who hitherto might not have paid much attention to these issues, might experience additional anxiety over and above those that already exist around the exploration of their presenting psychological problem.

To that extent, then, this therapeutic dyad could make available material which might be missed in other therapeutic pairings. There is an opportunity here, again, for this patient's whole self to be addressed in treatment, for intrapsychic issues to be dealt with in relation to the social construction of attitudes, ego functioning and personality. The race of the therapist will inescapably affect the therapy as it does when the therapist is white and the patient black. While the black psychotherapist in Britain would have had experience of working with (and having personal relationships with) white people, it might well be the case that the white patient is here for the first time making contact with a black person. The myths and fantasies that the white patient brings to the encounter will need to be worked through: 'When the therapist is a negro, certain important but little examined dynamic, economic and theoretical factors are introduced into an already complex inter/intra-psychic process. The very fact of the therapist being negro can modulate symbolic processes in the patient's mind which can have crucial effects upon the process of the therapy' (Curry, 1964).

The very effects encountered as a result of this therapeutic dyad can be denied or met with resistance in the patient. The symbols used by the patients, and the material of the dreams, will reveal elements of the repressed material. A white patient during the first months of therapy with a black male therapist reported a dream in which she was gradually becoming black. The physical transformation began at her head, the colour slowly working its way down to her toes. She reported her fear of not being recognised by her friends as the same person. This patient, whilst having been ambivalent about being in analytical therapy at the beginning, had now become very dependent on her therapist. She had a very poor sense of herself and her dream was related to her anxiety of merging with the therapist and losing her individuality – her whiteness among other things. This dream brought into the therapy her complex feelings about dependency and individuation as well as other themes. She had reported earlier that she 'did not notice' colour and indeed did not really notice that her therapist was black. The dream now freed her to say that, occasionally, when she came into the consulting room, she had an image of her therapist with a bone through his nose and a spear in his hand. The patient was upset about having to say this but said that she feared this preoccupation would get in the way if not reported. The material led the patient, several months later, to express her aggressive sexual wishes towards the therapist. She was eventually able to recognise the aggressive warrior in herself, which she had hitherto projected onto the black psychotherapist.

Some white patients who deny any difference between a black therapist and themselves, do so to preserve politeness and to secure against the seepage of unconscious material. Not responding to such politeness reveals anger and verbal attacks on the therapist in the usual way. These patients might not be able initially to consciously acknowledge their disappointment and rage at having a black therapist. The patients' 'politeness' robs them of the opportunity for such expression other than through the usual route of unconscious material, slips of the tongue, dreams, etc. The gloss of civility and education provides an overlay to mask what was previously learnt from society about black people. There is often a struggle for patients whose defences are watertight; they might deny the existence of and power of unconscious processes in other aspects of their lives. This transference, although one achieved through resistance, is a powerful one. The patients' psychic energies might be expended in the repressing of material, for example, in forgetting dreams and generally damming up the flow of material until the defences can no longer be maintained.

Case study

A white female patient began treatment with a black male therapist by stating that she did not believe in the unconscious. She ridiculed the therapist for 'believing in all of that nonsense about transference'. She constantly rejected interpretations: as a physical scientist, she saw therapy simply as a meeting of two people, one there to listen while the other bounced ideas around. She had been in analysis as a child and found it an entertaining way to spend her afternoons away from her school. Her reason for coming to therapy now was to help her clear up her ambivalence about getting married to her boyfriend and having babies. She had extensive social relations with both black and white people, and a sophisticated personal life in which active socialist politics played a large part.

For months this patient resisted interpretations of the transference until at one session when she presented her second dream. She dreamt that she was in the labour ward giving birth to her baby. She saw the midwife delivering a beautiful baby with black curly hair and wrapping it up in a blanket. On being brought the bundle, she looked into it and was shocked to see that it was not a baby at all but a little lump of shit. She told her therapist that she was very disappointed since all those months of waiting could not produce a real live baby. Following her associations, she revealed that she was first aware of her baby and of its being black. Once it had left her womb it became shit. She realised that the baby had something to do with her therapist and was very ashamed to admit this, feeling that she might offend him. She said that there must be something about the transference in the dream and for that reason was reluctant to bring the dream to therapy. The patient's aloofness about therapy, and the relationship with the therapist, subsequently changed. She has also been able to face her fear about not being able to produce a real live baby. Her resistance to the transference relationship with a black psychotherapist was also something to do with her resistance to produce her 'baby self' in the treatment.

White patients can also idealise their black therapist as one who has suffered and survived adversity. This unrealistic position often belies feelings of envy about the therapist as someone who appears to have escaped the oppression associated with being black in a white society. Any thoughts about the black therapist having 'sold out' will be repressed. The anger towards the therapist for having surmounted all obstacles represents a contrast with the patient who might feel that they should be equally secure and socially successful. Any doubts about the black therapist's credentials or actual ability could be masked by expressions of pleasure and admiration in the therapist as someone who could understand them because of their knowledge of suffering. The comment, 'I don't know what could have been worse, I could have had a black skin to contend with', is usually given sympathetically by such patients.

The black therapist brings his or her own history of relationships with white people to the treatment. White people would have been in positions of power and authority, both in the therapist's upbringing and professional training. The black psychotherapist, like anyone raised in a society which ascribes a stereotypical inferior position to black people, will have to work through this. While the trainee black psychotherapist has seldom if ever been able to escape the reality of racism by virtue of always having a black or brown skin, the subtle ways this is manifested in the therapeutic relationship have yet to be learned. The assumptions white patients bring to therapy about the superiority of whiteness and the inferiority of blackness will be largely hidden in symbols. Even when no obvious value is attached to colour, the patient's recognition of 'difference' will not always be easily accessible.

In treatment, the patients' assumed power by virtue of their whiteness has to be engaged in order to bring to consciousness the omnipotent and sometimes frightening fears of having power and control over the therapist. The black psychotherapist has the task of containing the white patient and their negative feelings. Patients with racist feelings which run particularly deeply often fear being 'found out' and evicted from therapy. This fear, related to the transference, can at times lead to them acting out in the work place or elsewhere with other black people. The therapist needs the confidence to stick to the analytic principles of illumination by interpretation.

In addition, the black psychotherapist needs to be very aware of the countertransference feelings of distancing themselves from patients who are seemingly abusive or racially demeaning. Collusive denial of difference can be motivated by the therapist's wish to 'keep things sweet'. The physical presence of the black psychotherapist will always affect the therapy and knowing when it is appropriate to pick this up from the patient's material will always be critical. Black therapists should not turn from this task for fear of their white patients accusing them of being too sensitive about their colour or of not having come to terms with their blackness. It must be remembered that the patient will use whichever means available to protect themselves from exposure and vulnerability and it is always their privilege to do so.

The black therapist and the black patient

As I have said, it is unlikely that a black psychotherapist in training will be offered theoretical or clinical material on the treatment of black and minority patients. Apart from the training analysis and the therapist's own personal experiences, the black candidate in training might be as ill-equipped to deal with the manifestations of racism in the consulting room as would be the white candidate. While training institutions have not addressed the particular issues that arise both in theory and technique for intercultural and inter-racial psychoanalytic treatment, the black therapist/black patient relationship is a complex one in that it also has to deal with the effects of racism. A black professional, raised in what is perceived as a racist society, will need to have acquired a positive self-identity against many odds. A positive identity will be one which resists the common negative and stereotyped views about black people. Some black patients might come to therapy not yet clear about this, harbouring a putative identity at a not-quite-conscious level. It should be expected that some patients will have the feeling of racial inferiority and that this will permeate their feelings about themselves. The black psychotherapist needs to have worked through this in the process of their own therapy in order to understand and help their subsequent patients. Even a black patient who has a sophisticated understanding of racism and its effect on the inner world might have a long-held fantasy of 'white as right'. The black therapist by his or her very presence in the consulting room presents a challenge to this view, one which the black patient has been brought up to believe.

A black patient's self-hatred will always provoke a powerful countertransference in the black psychotherapist. One response could be a nurturing concern, or a rejecting distance. The black therapist, who has already gone through this process, will always be reminded of their own pain if they had chosen to forget it. While the working through of feelings about 'whiteness' is not yet an issue in a white therapist/white patient relationship, feelings about 'blackness' are an inescapable part of the black patient/black therapist dyad. The black patient might have sought out a black psychotherapist in order to engage on a path of self-discovery with a particular intention of embracing their blackness in a safe place. Women psychotherapists, aware of the effects of sexism on the inner world, are sought out by women patients for similar reasons.

The black psychotherapist working in the public sector will often come across the black patient who feels that they have been 'cheated' by the institution by not being given a white therapist. Assuming that black by definition is 'not as good', the black patient feels that the clinic or hospital is uncaring, and indeed discriminating. The refusal in the black patient to see a black therapist as a professional of some worth, disguises their inner labyrinth of ego-related difficulties. The black patient, like the white patient, can perceive the black psythotherapist as inferior (or else someone who has sold out to white values). That a black person could aspire to and achieve professional status is, for them, a matter for questioning. For some black patients, professionalism would be equated with becoming 'like a white person' and enjoying economic and social privileges denied to them as black patients who belong in a different socio-economic group. While envy covers up the rejection and the ridicule, bringing this to the patient's awareness requires a great deal of care. The patient might vigorously deny envious feelings since the shame of exposure is linked, not just with failed achievement, but also with the patient's total experience of oppression and lack of opportunity. Hidden envy which is not brought out in the therapy will only perpetuate the patient's low self-image and impede development not only within the consulting room, but also outside it. Protecting the patient from the acknowledgement of their feelings of hatred or envy will be doing them a disservice.

Case study

A black female psychotherapist working in a state hospital was referred a young black woman who had been admitted after a breakdown. The patient had left home to attend university but had dropped out after the first term. She had been raised in an affluent suburb in a predominantly white provincial town. Her parents had themselves achieved professional and material success, one in law, the other in business. The patient avoided the other black patients on her ward and was silent during most of her sessions with the therapist. This contrasted with her lively, friendly relationships with white patients of her own age and with members of the white nursing staff.

The psychotherapist felt under some considerable pressure from her white colleagues to engage with this patient and make progress. There was also some reluctance to discharge the patient until something more was known about her, even though she would be able to attend for psychotherapy as an outpatient. The therapist had some difficulty in plucking up enough courage to bring into the session her concern that the patient had difficulties in feeling at ease with her, on account of her, the therapist's, blackness. The patient did not deny this. Bringing this out into the open was quite a relief since the patient was now free to talk about her upbringing, which she felt had not equipped her to feel confident about her colour. She had left a secure family and neighbourhood where she had safe white friends. Attending university in the city, she found it difficult to make friends and was very apprehensive about black people. She was depressed and isolated, feeling imprisoned at her university, not quite knowing who she was any more: looking black but feeling white.

In this case, treatment with a black therapist was akin to the patient holding up a mirror to herself. Her blackness was intertwined with her depression and subsequent breakdown, yet an understanding of this could have been missed in an assessment by a white professional. Similar difficulties in black children are usually more accessible for treatment. Black children raised in all-white caring institutions or families develop problems, to varying degrees, about their identity. Psychotherapy initially presents difficulties since these children often fear black people for what they represent. The children having hitherto denied or disregarded their blackness, the person of the black psychotherapist epitomises all that is bad and unwanted. With such children, therapy can only proceed with the collaboration of both a black and a white therapist.

The black psychotherapist, unlike the white psychotherapist, has to live in both a black world and a white world. It is possible for a white professional in Britain to have no social or personal relationships with black people. Black patients and therapists live in both settings and acquire the skills required to understand the subtlety and innuendo of both. The black therapist has the advantage of sharing some of the concerns and experience the black patient will bring. The way these experiences resonate in the inner world, and the way sense is made of them, provide the black therapist with a unique skill.

Chapter 10

Inner and Outer Reality in Children and Adolescents

CHRISO ANDREOU

> I am a little girl
> in a tiny world.
> My mother has gone and left me alone.
> I hate myself because I am black.
> I am going away to another world.
> Where someone can hold me in their arms,
> Surrounded by love, surrounded by charm.

This verse was written by Sherry, a 16-year-old girl in the course of long-term psychotherapy. At the time she wrote it, she was preoccupied with death and she reveals the pain of the abandoned and emotionally deprived child. The other, idealised, world of love and charm was Hades.

Before we can begin to think about the complex issue of racial and cultural identity we have to think about what is universally necessary for the individual self to survive and grow emotionally. Sherry expresses very vividly the pain caused by her emotional deprivation. Without 'good enough mothering', she remained emotionally a child that felt unloved and abandoned and who at times longed for death in order to stop feeling so much pain and loneliness. Without the internalisation of a 'good object' (in the first instance, the mother or mother substitute), the child cannot grow emotionally. Winnicott and Bion (1963) have described the necessary environmental, emotional and mental states of the mother that are needed for growth.

I begin with the need to think about deprivation and severe emotional disturbance because the majority of children and adolescents referred to the Nafsiyat Centre (see Chapter 2) are referred through the Social Services. Often social workers will have put thought and time into trying to make available black adults as foster parents or residential social workers to enable the children to identify with and relate to adults from their own race and cultural group. Their hope is that through these new relationships the children would begin to heal some of their own wounds and confusion about themselves. It is difficult for these workers to face the fact that this is often not enough, or worse, that such model figures can be rejected.

Sometimes the emotions aroused by these children in the social workers are unbearable, making them feel desperate and useless. The children's and adolescents' expression of anger and rejection have an additional dimension: unlike white children in care, they also reject their own culture and race or identify negatively with it, at times experiencing disgust at the colour of their skins. At times this arouses such primitive anxieties in the social workers, that their referral to Nafsiyat is not just a recognition that these children need psychotherapy but that they themselves, as white workers, feel there is nothing they can do; they do not understand what is happening and they are unable to think; this is expressed in the referral through such statements as, 'thinks she is white'; 'needs a black therapist or counsellor'.

The Nafsiyat Centre was the chosen agency for referral because it was perceived in the first instance as a place where, to quote one worker, 'cultural and racial factors would be taken into consideration'. The hidden, seldom verbalised, reasons and fantasies were revealed when we discussed the clients with the referring agency. Nafsiyat thus became a place for white referrers to discuss their own confused and painful feelings, their own helplessness and guilt at not being, according to their own lights, 'good enough' – feelings which were aroused in them by the children. So these workers came searching for a place or a person who would be for them the representations of the necessary adult/parent figure that would help them: the therapist from the same racial or cultural group. In fact they needed an idealised parent who could heal the wounds of these children, expressing clearly the children's own need in the first instance for the original 'good object'.

The white social workers were unable to avoid feeling uncomfortable and often said that they felt guilty or that they felt 'they represented the oppressive racist society'. The black social workers who referred to the Centre expressed a wish to protect and repair the damage done to these children and again emphasised the importance of having a black therapist with whom the child or adolescent would identify and thereby gain their own racial identity and ego strength that would protect them and help them fight expressions of racism in the world outside without the fear of disintegration of the self.

The sad truth is that no one can simply construct for themselves 'an identity'. Culture is both inherited and has to be recreated through experience so that it may reside within the individual in memory and feeling. It is the product of experience and history represented in individuals through our internalised parents and by the values and traditions they have passed on to us. Ethnic minority children are born into a society which often differs markedly in its social and family organisation and they themselves may experience different types of care and upbringing.

The work of Erikson (1968) and Kakar (1970) shows evidence that cultural factors in upbringing have an impact on the development of the personality and may reinforce or suppress certain specific internal conflicts. They may stimulate the use of certain types of defence mechanisms, or suppress others, in this way making the expression of certain behaviour culture-specific as well as influencing object representation and object relations.

A girl brought up in a white foster home told me, 'I thought I was white until one day I heard my foster mother say in a whisper to a friend, "she *is* black"'. After hearing this, she went to the bathroom and tried to scrape her skin white. This physical experience of identity through skin is a theme which continually recurs in therapy with black children. How it is dealt with – the theme of feeling different/being different – is the focus of my discussion in the following case examples; the individual who 'feels different' and who comes from a culture where people are devalued and rejected because of the colour of their skin will always have to face questions about their identity in relation to the others. In therapy this has to be dealt with in what is known as the transference and countertransference.

Racism and cultural difference in the transference

Case study

Hussein was seven years old when he was referred for therapy by his school. The school was concerned by his lack of progress, his inability to make friends, and his tendency to regress in class and become rather babyish and 'switched off'. His parents had been living in England for several years, spoke no English, and lived and worked among their closely knit community. They were very concerned about their son and felt lost and bewildered as to how to help him.

I will use some of the case material from the beginning of his therapy to illustrate how cultural differences arose in the transference and which, I think, was particularly important in engaging this boy and helping him feel understood rather than alienated. In doing this, I am aware I am being selective, not illustrating fully all aspects of his personality and the problems of his emotional development. Emphasising just a part of the transference does not mean that this aspect is what I hold most important but I do feel it brings into focus a conflict which is certainly real and is an everyday reality for children from ethnic minorities in Britain.

In the first session Hussein was evidently preoccupied about my origins. He looked at me curiously and told me: 'you are not Turkish but you are not English' and demanded to know where I came from. I took this up with him by saying that it felt very important that he knew where I came from and what kind of a person I was. Was I going to be someone that would understand what it feels like to be Turkish but born in this country? To understand how difficult it is sometimes to know where he himself comes from? And where he belongs?

He looked at me seriously and then said that at school sometimes they call him 'Paki' – he looked down at his hands (he was a dark boy) and he shouted at them that he is not a 'Paki'; those boys are nasty to 'Pakis', they hurt them. He doesn't like boys, they are so aggressive; his best friend at school is a girl. I replied that he was not sure yet what or who I was. 'Am I going to be aggressive and hurt him? Not listen when he tells me he is Turkish? Confuse him with the other children I see, maybe Pakistani children?'

This boy was unusually open and he verbalised his anxieties about me: I represented someone alien to him which aroused anxieties about his own feelings of being an outsider, a victim of discrimination, and his confusion at being a Turkish child brought up in England. What I represented in the transference had to develop slowly and would change from one session to another. I was not Turkish like his parents therefore I was not represented as a parental figure; the outside world made him suspicious and frightened.

As a transference developed he became more trusting and more talkative. He told me that he suffered from asthma. He went into hospital often. He was jealous of his 18-month-old brother and sometimes he felt like hitting him. That frightened him. His fear of his own aggression was often projected onto other boys at school, often made him keep away from them, and instead he only wanted to play with girls. He talked of his best friend Joanne, an English girl. He had never visited an English home. (He didn't want to anyway – English mothers feed their children bad food and when the children grow up they throw them out.) I interpreted that he saw me as the English mother who sometimes feeds the small Hussein part of him with bad food and that he was frightened that if he grew up I would throw him out and would not want to see him any more.

It is interesting to note here that the primitive splitting of the good, present, feeding mother and the bad, deserting and depriving mother is divided by nationalities. Difference in cultures can be a good vehicle into which our split bad feelings and good feelings are projected. This is also used, of course, by the parents of children to safeguard their own sense and idealisation of their own culture. The more frightened and threatened a minority culture feels from the majority culture the more protective and enclosed it becomes, keeping the 'bad' (i.e. English) influence outside.

The question of loyalty to parents and their values is more obviously common with adolescent conflicts than with those of younger children. With ethnic minority children, however, it has to be borne in mind that it is always present. For a Muslim boy like Hussein, in therapy, the topic may be brought up in a session, as in the session where he was building a farm. He gathered together the family of toy pigs. He picked one up and caressed it gently and said that he liked piggies. Having said that, he looked at me anxiously and said that he shouldn't like pigs because he is Turkish; his mother told him that pigs are not nice, they are dirty. 'You shouldn't kill animals,' he says; he doesn't like to eat them; he doesn't want to kill them either as long as pigs don't make 'a mess'. I interpreted his unconscious fear of his own aggression and 'pigginess', which reduced his anxiety, and then explored with him what he thought his mother meant when she said he was Turkish and he must not like pigs.

I was, of course, aware of the religious aspect to all this but as a therapist my role was not to dismiss, question or – worse – reassure him that he was certainly not being disloyal to his parents, but to reduce his anxiety and help him to go back and talk to his parents further about this aspect of his religion and what it meant. I feel that this needed to be explored for he would surely come to know that other children at school eat pork and certainly didn't see it as dirty or disgusting. Unless children are helped to understand their culture so that they can identify positively through 'knowing' it experientially, they will face unnecessary conflicts with the therapist's values.

Case study

The next case is of a six-year-old West Indian boy who was referred by the local Social Services. He had been in and out of 'Care' since he was a baby and now had returned to his mother once again in the hope that this time, with support and therapy for both mother and child, they could stay together. His mother was very young, and had herself been brought up in Care. She suffered from depression and felt unable to cope with Leroy's demand on her. She only wanted her son to behave himself and be grown up.

Leroy, when I started to see him, would often want to be a baby in sessions, desperate for love and attention. He was very puzzled and hurt by his last removal from his foster home where he had been for two years. He felt he had done something wrong, he must have been bad or they didn't like him because he was black (his foster parents were white). Being black and what it meant to him was a theme which frequently came into sessions. His mother herself felt unhappy about her colour and would often express the opinion that no one had helped her or wanted her because she was black. Children often represent again for their parents how they think of themselves. Leroy identified with his rejected black mother and saw himself as another rejected black baby whom nobody wanted.

He came into the room and sat at his table, smiled at me, looked inside his box (containing toys and pencils which are usually provided for children in therapy) and checked to see that everything was still there since the last time. I suggested that he was checking to see if I had kept his things safe and not given anything away or allowed any other child to play with them.

He took out some brown plasticine and proceeded to mould a baby. When he had finished he held it up for me to look at, 'look a brown baby, I am brown, here, take it'. I took it and interpreted that he was giving me the baby part of himself to hold and maybe to mother.

He took the 'baby' from my hand and sat it down on the table. He started to giggle to himself. I wondered what he was thinking about. He looked at me shyly, then he said, 'pooh is brown, shitty baby, naughty baby'. Then he grimaced and told me that he didn't like going to the toilet. When I explored this with him he said that he imagined that spiders would crawl out of the toilet and bite his bottom. 'Disgusting', he said to the brown baby, 'you did a pooh-pooh'. Then he made a sound as if he was drinking and said the baby is disgusting, drinking its pee-pee. I said that during our separation from one week to another the baby part of him is left without the good breast that feeds him with good milk and leaves him alone, thirsty, with only horrible urine to drink.

'I am frightened of breast, I think the breast is like a lion that would eat me up'. I said that when the good breast is not available to the baby Leroy, he gets very angry and attacks the good breast and those thoughts frighten him because he then imagines that the breast becomes a lion that would eat him up instead. He smiled and said that the baby was a baby 'Miss Andreou'. I said that now I have to be the baby that feels left alone and hungry with only its urine to drink so that I know what it feels like.

He became preoccupied with modelling another baby with the plasticine. 'White, clumsy, thin', he was speaking in a baby voice, 'I do not want to be a baby, I want to be a grown up'. I interpreted his fear of feeling small and vulnerable and his wish to be a grown up seven-year-old.

He finished the baby and came and placed it on my desk and told me that the brown baby was for me to take home. I said that he wanted me to keep the baby part of himself to take home and be looked after by me. He was letting me know that the baby part feels neglected and abandoned during the time that I am not around; he needs looking after all the time not for just an hour a week. He said that he forgot what I looked like when he didn't see me. I disappeared from his mind. Perhaps he thought I forgot all about him during the week.

He started modelling: what he made me was a basket and he was going to fill it with lovely food. He took a piece of brown plasticine and he said it was chocolate – chocolate was lovely, did I like chocolate? Then he made a milk bottle so that the baby would have milk. He told me that I must feed the baby from the milk bottle. He then brought the second baby and put it next to the brown baby 'Miss Andreou' and instructed me that I must feed them until next week.

There was a shift in the session from the colour brown representing a brown fecal baby (the shitty baby, pooh baby) drinking its urine, to brown representing good food (chocolate). Children's experience of colour will represent different things at different times. Sometimes in a case it will depend on the level of emotional development. At a very primitive level, thinking becomes very concrete and the process of symbolisation can break down. Once his deeper feelings are interpreted (and thus contained), his anxiety having been reduced, his thinking moved on from concrete to the symbolic: in this case through bad feelings to good feelings, from being a brown fecal baby drinking urine, to a baby needing to drink milk and needing sweet brown chocolate.

Issues of identification

Case study

Yvonne was 15 years old when she was referred for psychotherapy by her social worker. She was at the time living in a Children's Home and the staff were worried by her depression, violent outbursts, and the fact that she wanted to be white. Although she was in contact with her parents, she regarded them as 'low life'. Her carers felt her behaviour to be strange. She was unable to make friends or close relationships and made people feel uncomfortable around her.

Yvonne came from a large West Indian family and was the youngest of eight children. She was sexually abused in childhood by a relative and ran away from home at the age of 11. She was regarded as 'beyond parental control' and was received into the care of the Local Authority. Attempts to foster her had failed as she would not consider a black family, or indeed anyone who was not rich, middle-class and living outside London.

When she began therapy she presented herself as a young girl who was struggling very hard to present herself to the outside world as someone that was sophisticated, grown up, and who knew her own mind. She lived in a fantasy world where things and people were very good and perfect (this she associated with the white middle-class) or else very bad and 'low life' (this is where she placed black people and her own family).

Such splitting of external reality into good and bad is a mechanism of defence which Yvonne used to defend herself against her pain, confusion and fear of annihilation. To illustrate this I will refer to an incident from her therapy.

Yvonne came to one session very tense and angry. Sitting down in her chair she told me that she had had a row with one of the residential social workers. 'How I hate them all, it's shitty being in Care, they still haven't found me a school'. They expect her to have another tutor. She is fifteen and she cannot read or write: what is going to happen to her? She felt that they looked at her and saw that she was a healthy fifteen-year-old and because she told them she can look after herself they don't look beyond that.

I suggested that she saw me too as someone that didn't look beyond what she looks like on the outside; that I too thought she could manage. I was not capable of realising that inside she felt small and vulnerable and needed looking after by a mother who finds her a school and helps her to grow up and be able to look after herself. She appeared to be far away, not taking in what I was saying. I pointed this out to her and she told me that, that is how she is when she feels angry: 'in one ear out of the other' and continued to tell me that her nephew who is only six can read better than she can; when she was young she used to hide the fact that she could not read. She thought it started when she was eight years old and started to have problems at home. Nobody at school bothered to ask her why, they just said that she was naughty, no one asked her why she looked a mess. She felt no one knows or can understand what she has been through. She ran away from home when she was only eleven. She lived rough, she knows what street life is all about. She had a friend who was in Care too but is now eighteen and has her own flat, but it was kept in a disgusting state, filthy; her own room is always neat and tidy.

I interpreted her fear that unless she finds someone to help her she will be just like her friend, eighteen, grown up and living in a disgusting state. 'Black people are dirty', she said in a disgusted way. Just because she likes nice clothes and wants the good things in life, like a nice house, and wants to live outside London, they say she is a white girl.

She was terrified; she identified with this friend of hers living in a disgusting state which so reflected her own internal state of mind of being in a mess that she projected it outward. When I asked her whether it was really true that black people were dirty and whether the good things in life were not also their desire and pointed out that in fact in reality they could also have them if they were in a position to do so, she nodded when I differentiated her fantasies and how she mixed up fantasy with reality. I then interpreted that she imagined I thought she was a 'black disgusting girl'. She nodded and began to talk about sexual abuse and how that has left her feeling dirty and disgusting, that no washing could ever take the feeling away.

The girl's feeling of disgust and mess was often projected onto the outside. Since society often degrades black people and their way of life, she has learned to do so as well. As a white therapist, she feared that I would touch on the feelings which were so hidden underneath. When I did she would not listen. Her feelings of disgust about her skin were due to sexual abuse and she preferred to keep them at bay by keeping them skin deep as she often wanted therapy to be at that level also.

This girl highlights the crucial issue of the nature of identification. That of a person who takes up a negative identification to her race and origins. Part can be seen to reflect white society's view of that race, but to rely purely on sociological terms about racism in therapy is of little use. Our concern is with the internal state of the young persons involved and how we can help them move on from that negative split to a more positive identification.

Erikson (1968) defines the quest for individuality as a process located both in the core of the individual and also in their communal culture. This girl had no core: she lacked a good internal object inside which she would need to gain before she could feel rooted.

A summary of racism and cultural differences in the transference

(1)   What does the therapist represent at a particular moment in a session for the child?
(2)   Is there anxiety and confusion about colour or race aroused by the outside world?
(3)   How is that represented in the child's internal world?
(4)   Is there confusion of customs and beliefs with home and the majority culture? (This needs to be explored and understood rather than pathologised.)
(5)   Attack on racial identity from the outside has to be acknowledged and believed as a reality rather than interpreted as an unconscious process which can only lead to more persecution and feelings of alienation.
(6)   The therapist in the transference will not always represent the internal parents but others from the outside world such as teachers or anyone from the majority culture.
(7)   The children or the family's grievance might be connected in the reality of prejudice, racism and disadvantage.
(8)   Feelings aroused in the countertransference will be very strong and there is always the danger of not being able to think, to stick with the differences, to bear not knowing and becoming 'the bad other' in the transference.

Chapter 11

Intercultural Social Work

ELAINE ARNOLD

In the UK today there are many groups of people who differ ethnically and culturally from the majority population. Some of this majority population, perhaps themselves lacking self esteem, hold negative attitudes and perceptions of minorities. Attitudes influence behaviour. Dismissive and rejecting behaviour towards ethnic minority groups tends to undermine the self-image of individuals, and to foster feelings of inferiority among their more vulnerable members.

Ideally, people develop a sense of well-being through their positive interaction with others in day-to-day experiences; it is not surprising that those who feel themselves marginal to their society, who live their lives in the shadow of a dichotomised 'we' and 'they', who are victims of subtle prejudice and at times overt racism, may sometimes succumb. When an individual from any ethnic group experiences a stressful situation through the breakdown of interpersonal relationships, help may be sought from social workers in the health or social services, from voluntary agencies or from those in private practice, especially if traditional support is unavailable (whether this comprises the nuclear or extended family, the religious adviser or the neighbourhood community).

Social workers who work with ethnic minorities are themselves not immune from prejudiced attitudes and perceptions; as Klineberg (1982) puts it, they may have pictures in their heads that give the impression that 'we' (as social workers) know what 'they' are like even before we have actually met them.

Both social workers and clients bring to their interaction certain values acquired during socialisation within their own backgrounds. Frequently the workers fail to recognise that clients from minority racial groups may have suffered previously unpleasant or belittling experiences at the hands of other professionals in health, welfare, housing or education agencies, experiences which may influence their more current meeting. Perlman (1979) points out that when the consequences of conscious and unconscious feelings and attitudes about others that we carry with us from earlier relationships occur as transferences and countertransferences in the therapeutic encounter, they create a particularly charged situation. The 'they all look alike' attitude which is frequently expressed about black people may similarly be applied by black clients towards white workers. It is important that the worker is able to anticipate this phenomenon and to deal with it in order to build a satisfactory working relationship.

Specific knowledge of the client population always contributes to the effectiveness of a social worker. Many white professionals who wish to work 'interculturally' live in social isolation from the minority ethnic groups; their only experience of these groups is when individuals are under stress. There is then no way to decide how different the client's behaviour and experiences are from those accepted within his or her group, or what assets are available within the community. Negative stereotypical images about the client's family organisation, choice of partners, and child rearing practices, derived from moments of dysfunction, become the basis for everyday knowledge. Not surprisingly, the outcome of the interaction is frequently viewed with pessimism.

Additionally, the client who comes from an ethnic group different from that of the social worker, may leave the latter deskilled by objecting that if he or she were black, or of the same cultural background, the problems would certainly be better understood. In this respect the client seems to share the view of the anthropologist Patricia King (1982) who holds that racial differences always affect the rapport between workers and client, while cultural differences reduce the worker's ability to understand the nature of the client's problem. It is important that the social worker disentangles him- or herself from implicit racial and cultural stereotypes in careful interviewing in order to establish the needs of particular clients within their own terms, and by demonstrating competence, genuineness and empathic understanding in order to gain the client's confidence and trust.

Many white social workers admit to anxieties of 'not being accepted by the client', of 'being called racist', 'not being able to understand', or 'not being understood' or 'the client perceiving their questioning as official prying' when a knowledge of family relationships is necessary. They are worried they will either over-react or under-react, especially when working with mental illness or child abuse. Sometimes these fears and anxieties may be so great that the worker is effectively paralysed and fails to help the client in any way. Appropriate supervision, in which the worker is able to analyse and articulate their perceptions and feelings about race and about culture, and how these affect practice, is vitally important. There are times when those social workers who are themselves immigrants, may find the pain of clients from minority groups mirrored within themselves, and may identify so closely that they are unable to be useful. This too indicates the need for sensitive and aware supervision.

Social workers need to recognise when the specific problems with which the client is struggling are exacerbated by the following: the unexpressed grief and mourning which comes from separation and from missing the support of relatives and friends due to emigration; overwhelmingly poor economic circumstances; deficiencies within the material environment such as inadequate housing; the effects of racial disadvantage, especially the experience of being marginal to our society, the sense of not belonging; economic exploitation on the basis of race or gender; the experience of the young living within 'two cultures'; the emotional conflicts of adolescents as they struggle to reconcile their inner and outer worlds.

When working interculturally, the genuine anxiety we have about working empathetically with people from different backgrounds is exaggerated. The following responses of some white social workers in a training seminar to a case study exercise are not atypical.

Case study

A 14-year-old black girl was referred for assessment with complaints by teachers of persistent truancy. On the occasions when she attended, she was very disruptive, talking incessantly and interrupting the teacher, refusing to pay attention to any instruction, and encouraging her peers to join her in her escapades. Her parents had admitted that they were unable to control her difficult behaviour at home and were afraid that she would influence her younger siblings.

Asked for their initial responses to this case on reading the referral, answers included the following:
'Hmm, trouble.'
'If West Indian, perhaps her parents were too strict.'
'If Indian or Pakistani, perhaps parents were arranging a marriage for her.'
Repeating the exercise on another occasion with the same referral now being of a white girl, responses were:
'Adolescent acting out.'
'May be influenced by peer group.'
'Struggling for independence and resenting the responsibility of looking after her younger siblings.'
Asked then to examine the differences in response, the social workers were taken aback to realise that they had not thought about the usual developmental problems of adolescence in relation to the black girl. Studying the difference in their reactions, social workers felt they had been influenced by the client being black, in responding to an image of black children as inevitable

failures at school, and in trying to recall some of the information gathered from various sources about the 'culture' and child rearing practices of the group to which the girl probably belonged: West Indian 'Victorian discipline'; arranged marriages.

Similar exercises can be useful in training workers of different backgrounds to examine the ways their stereotypes can affect policy decisions, and to facilitate their own use of social work theory in practice with all client groups. They also serve as a guard against lumping together all people from a particular racial or cultural group and against failing to perceive the client as a unique individual.

In working across ethnic groups, it is vital to maintain a balance between not overlooking our shared and universal human characteristics and needs, attributing all the client's problems to some 'cultural' peculiarity on the one hand, and on the other, neglecting cultural variability with the aim of treating everyone the same. There is a danger of selecting what may seem a 'positive' characteristic of a particular cultural group as the single significant solution for making a decision in an intricate case. This was illustrated in the tragic example of Tyra Henry who died as a result of physical abuse by her father. While it is true that there certainly is a tradition of African–Caribbean grandmothers playing an active and successful role in caring for their grandchildren, in this case neither the social and economic constraints, nor the emotional state of the particular grandmother, were taken into account.

Tyra had been placed to live with her maternal grandmother who was living in substandard accommodation for which she was in rent arrears. The electricity had been cut off for non-payment of bills. Grandmother was suffering from severe stress due to several recent major losses – her previous accommodation had been destroyed by a fire which had also claimed the life of her son; her husband had died after a short illness; her grandson had been severely damaged through physical abuse and had been adopted. It was therefore unlikely that it would have been possible for Mrs Henry to be the idealised coping carer for an active young child.

In the subsequent report 'Whose Child? The Report of the Public Inquiry into the Death of Tyra Henry' (1987), it was recommended that this problem of 'positive' stereotypes needed to be fully considered. Pinderhughes (1983), discussing the empowerment of social work clients and social workers themselves, draws attention to the need for focusing simultaneously on the realities of the outer world of the individual and their families, as well as on how they manage the situation. While this is relevant for working with all families, it is especially important for clients belonging to groups who are disadvantaged by discrimination on the basis of race or class, or through being single parent families. She stresses that 'knowing how power and powerlessness operate in human systems is a key to effective intervention. Strategies based on this knowledge offer both client and worker an opportunity for constructive management of powerlessness on individual, familial and social systems levels'.

Illness and distress

People of Asian, African or African–Caribbean origins may not identify a physical problem as something sufficiently serious to warrant a formal examination by a doctor, but at the same time they may be aware that they are not 'coping' as well as they could in other areas. Since there are now increasing numbers of community facilities – Drop-In Centres and Counselling Services – people are beginning perhaps to feel less inhibited in discussing their mental and physical health with a stranger. Social workers in these centres can be of immense help in promoting an understanding of 'mental health as a condition of the whole personality – an outgrowth of one's total life, promoted or hindered by the day-to-day experiences and not only by major crises'.

Robertson (1977) carried out work among a London group of mothers of West Indian origin who had been reunited with their children after having left them behind in the West Indies for varying periods. She found that a third of the mothers who had unsatisfactory relationships with their children upon reunion also complained of indifferent physical health and suffered somatic anxiety. Their most frequent complaints were indigestion, headaches and backaches; some did not specify a pain in any part of the body, only a general malaise and, although they did not associate their complaints with stress, worry or anxiety, these were certainly found to be present on questioning. For example 'Mrs Hill' complained of constant indigestion and pains in her stomach, but subsequently revealed her anxiety over her only daughter who was not progressing satisfactorily at school. Mrs Hill herself had been deprived of education since her own mother died when she was very young and her stepmother had kept her at home whilst sending her own children to school. She recollected this treatment with growing resentment as she realised her inability to help her own daughter. She had never been able to tell anyone of her resentment before.

Family conflict

Family conflict and its subsequent personal unhappiness occur in all cultures. How families are helped to resolve these will depend on how social workers and other professionals relate to values other than their own. Indeed 'any social worker must be aware of the relativity of his or her own values in relation to the values of the person, group or community with whom they work. A sensitive training programme will provide opportunities to reconsider their assumptions, methods of work and values, in relation to different races and cultures' (CCETSW, 1983). Like the case studies in the Appendix, the following example has been useful in such training sessions:

Case study

Mrs Clarke, before she emigrated to England, had lived in a small rural village in one of the islands in the Caribbean together with her common-law husband, Errol Andrews, and their two daughters. When the girls, Beryl and Diane, were nine and five years old, Errol left her to marry someone else. Mrs Clarke placed the children in the care of Errol's mother (her own parents were both dead) and set off to the town to find a job, and to get away from the painful presence of her ex-partner with his new wife. She formed a relationship with a Mr Barker who soon left for England and asked her to join him after five years. They married and settled down in Bradford, but after two years the marriage broke down and Mrs Clarke moved to London to be near friends and Errol's sister's family, the Warners, who were already living there. Consciously or unconsciously, Mrs Clarke tried to gain support from this extended family. She was housed by the local council in a one-bedroom flat but, planning for a reunion with her daughters, she applied for larger accommodation and was placed on a housing list for this. She worked in a local factory and faithfully sent remittances for the support of the children.

For three years Mrs Clarke tried unsuccessfully to obtain permission for the girls to join her. She was finally able to convince Home Office officials that as a single parent she had demonstrated a continuing financial and personal interest by sending letters, presents and money for the children's upkeep. Diane was allowed to join her. The older daughter, Beryl, now eighteen, was required to apply in her own right as she was not considered dependent on her mother. Mrs Clarke was overjoyed when Diane, now fourteen, arrived. For the first few months, in spite of the cramped living accommodation, their relationship was a loving and happy one. Mother and daughter were together. As time went by the problems started. Diane was encouraged to rebel against her mother's 'old fashioned' lifestyle by her paternal aunt, Mrs Warner, and her cousins. They had long accommodated to inner-city London life and were critical of Mrs Clarke whose 'restricted' life seemed to centre around the church. Mrs Warner encouraged Diane to stay over in her home during the afternoons, after school and then at weekends.

Mrs Clarke, with her strong work ethic, expected Diane to return home after school, do her homework, and then help in preparing the evening meal, to be an economic and emotional support to her when she returned after a hard day's work for them both. One evening Mrs Clarke forbade Diane to go to her aunt's for a party. Diane insisted she would go. In the argument which ensued, Mrs Clarke slapped her. Diane did remain at home that evening but on the following day put together all her belongings and moved into her aunt's house. Mrs Clarke expected that after a few days Diane would regret her decision and return home, or even that her aunt would insist that she did so. Neither happened. Diane remained with her aunt. Fraught with maternal concern, with the knowledge of her responsibilities for Diane, but too angry with Mrs Warner to go to her house, Mrs Clarke, very hurt, went along to the school to enlist the help of Diane's teacher. She talked incessantly, was tearful, and was unable to communicate her position clearly to the teacher. The latter referred her to a social worker and Mrs Clarke overheard the telephone conversation in which the teacher described her as 'mad'. She did, however, go to the social services agency, where the young white social worker seemed to identify with Diane and her wish for 'independence'; worse, she was reluctant to consider Mrs Clarke and Diane together as a 'family'. Not being helped there, Mrs Clarke referred herself to an intercultural counselling agency (Nafsiyat).

Questions to be asked about the social worker

What was the white social worker's understanding of this African–Caribbean family and its pattern of child rearing (especially relevant as the child had only recently joined her mother who was clinging to her traditional ways)? What was her theoretical knowledge about the experience of separation and loss, and how did she relate it to both Mrs Clarke and Diane? What was her knowledge of adolescent development and did she apply this to Diane? How aware was the social worker of Mrs Clarke's own needs for nurturing, of her need to achieve a successful relationship with a loved one since most of her previous relationships had failed? Were the social worker's values inducing her to think of Mrs Warner's family as 'normal' and acceptable, as she herself was married and living with her husband and children, in contrast to Mrs Clarke's one-parent family? How judgemental was the social worker being? How realistic were her fears of Mrs Clarke physically abusing Diane? Was Mrs Clarke's own understanding explored? Were her intentions to physically punish Diane an attempt to exercise control, or to communicate her own frustration? Did the social worker acknowledge the mother's legal responsibility for her daughter? Diane's rights and her mother's rights did not coincide – what attempts could be made to reconcile these?

Questions to be asked about Mrs Clarke

Was Mrs Clarke taking the social worker as some sort of maternal authority figure who would sort everything out for her? Or did she find difficulty in relating to this worker who seemed so much younger than herself? Did she know the social worker was married? What did she think the social worker thought of her?

Some policy issues

Had inadequate housing exacerbated the problems between the mother and an adolescent girl who had no privacy? Would Mrs Clarke have been more adequately helped by a social worker of a similar race and cultural background? Were there any such people within this social service agency? Had the social worker's training been one to fit her for work with a multicultural and multiracial caseload? Was her supervisor able to help her?

The Social Services Inspectorate has recently suggested to Directors of Social Services in Britain that, 'Social Services must address and seek to meet the needs of children and family from all groups in the community' (Utting, 1990). Because of demography, social workers from the majority population would tend to work with black and minority ethnic groups. Social workers who themselves come from minority groups would not be expected to work only in special areas and only with clients of their own background. It was argued that the provision of services which could reach all members of the community called for the development within Social Services Departments of awareness, sensitivity, understanding of the different cultures of groups in the local community, and an understanding of the material and psychological effects of racial discrimination on these groups. Necessary experience and expertise would be provided in the staffing services and through consultative relationships with other professions and services and with the community (Utting, 1990).

The action which follows this directive will indicate how seriously intercultural social work is accepted throughout the country. Those social workers from intercultural agencies like Nafsiyat, who work intensively for shorter periods, and with smaller caseloads, and who are well supervised, are in a strong position to help develop effective intercultural practice, and to take up the opportunities for sharing their experience and expertise for the benefit of both clients and colleagues.

Chapter 12

Therapeutic Approaches With Survivors of Torture

STUART TURNER

In the 1980s, torture was being practised systematically by one in every three countries (Amnesty International, 1984) thereby constituting one of the largest preventable causes of physical and psychological morbidity in the modern world. A massive personal trauma, it occurs within a violent socio-political context and affects healthy people. For survivors, existence often becomes filled with bitter memories both of personal pain and of witnessed tragedy. In this chapter, some of the common psychological reactions and approaches to therapy, informed by cultural and political as well as by psychological processes, will be described.

Torture and other forms of organised state violence

Torture has been defined as 'systematic and deliberate infliction of acute pain in any form by one person on another . . . in order to accomplish the purpose of the former against the will of the latter' (Amnesty International, 1975). It is not the quasi-judicial inquisition of earlier centuries, when guilt rested on confession, and torture was considered to be a more or less acceptable way of obtaining this, the 'queen' of proofs. It has become in the twentieth century, a tool of repression, denied in the double-talk of state authorities yet widely employed against target groups or communities (Rasmussen, 1990). The United Nations (1984) has explicitly clarified the subject role of the state by including in its definition a clause that torture is (always) '. . . inflicted by or at the instigation of or with the consent of a public official or other person acting in an official capacity'. Of course, it is not just the individual who suffers. For every person tortured, there will be family or friends, colleagues, and political, ethnic or religious associates who are also touched by the experience.

It is possible to list some of the common forms of torture. In a recent review of the (openly published) scientific literature, Goldfeld *et al.* (1988), found that beating, kicking, threats, humiliation, electrical torture, blindfolding, mock execution, being made to witness other people being tortured, 'submarino' torture[1], isolation, starvation, sleep deprivation, suspension, sexual torture including rape of men and women, burning and 'falaka'[2] were among the most frequently recorded techniques. The deficiencies of this sort of analysis are obvious. It is a catalogue of tragedy, yet fails to offer a sense of the meaning of these events to the individuals concerned.

Jacobo Timerman, in his writing, gives a personal insight into one aspect of the trauma experience. 'Nothing can compare to those family groups that were tortured, often together, sometimes separately, but in view of one another or in different cells, while one was aware of the other being tortured. The entire affective world, constructed over the years with utmost difficulty, collapses with a kick in the father's genitals, a smack on the mother's face, an obscene insult to the sister or the sexual violation of a daughter. Suddenly an entire culture based on familial love, devotion, the capacity for mutual sacrifice, collapses. Nothing is possible in such a universe, and that is precisely what the torturers know' (Timerman, 1981). For many, the worst experience is this powerlessness to protect other people, even young children, from torture.

Some talk about the firing squad to which they were taken with other prisoners, and how, following the report of the guns, there was the slow realisation that, surrounded by death, they had been deliberately allowed to survive, that this was just another part of the torture.

Close proximity to death (of self and of others) is a common theme in torture. In submarino torture, for example, the person's head is forced under water, often foul water, and held there until the urge to breathe can no longer be resisted. At the point of inhaling water or even after losing consciousness, the head is just as quickly removed. Usually consciousness returns, but with the awareness that the whole terrifying procedure will be repeated.

Torture has been described as the perversion of an intimate relationship (Schlapobersky and Bamber, 1988). It is a personalised attack, carried out to achieve specific changes using techniques chosen for each individual, bearing in mind his or her social and cultural environment. Thus the personal meaning of sexual torture of women becomes more apparent when it is appreciated that in many communities, rape carries a stigma for the survivor which may lead to rejection, even expulsion from the social group. For some women, it is impossible to admit that they have been detained at all, because this would lead to their being cast out on the likely assumption that they had been raped. At the time when they most need the support of friends, they are prevented by shame and fear from asking.

The pain of torture may be physical or psychological, yet the purpose of torture is always to have a psychological effect on individuals and usually to exert a political effect on communities or even whole countries. With an understanding of these primarily oppressive and repressive aims, a strict definition of torture in terms of characteristic injuries or techniques becomes largely irrelevant outside a narrow medico-legal arena. Torture commonly takes place within a hostile socio-political climate, for example with 'disappearances', death squads, and wide-scale repression of a target group. A more helpful terminology, therefore, is to include all these within a broader category of 'organised state violence'. In this way, it is the purpose of the activity, and hence its usual effects, which become of fundamental importance.

Torture and refuge

Torture affects not only people in countries where torture takes place. For many survivors, the only way to manage the experience is to seek safety outside the country of violence. A refugee has been defined by another United Nations resolution as a person who, 'owing to a well founded fear of being persecuted for reasons of race, religion, nationality, membership of a particular social group or political opinion, is outside the country of his nationality and is unable or, owing to such fear, is unwilling to avail himself of the protection of that country'. In the world today it is estimated that there are 12–15 million refugees (see, for example, Andreassen, 1989) with relatively few (about 700 000) in Europe. However, whether they remain in their original country, escape into a neighbouring state to possibly end up in a large refugee camp, or enter a more remote country, many torture survivors will have high levels of distress. It is a sad truth that all too often the experiences in the country of refuge only add to their problems.

Individual psychological reactions to torture

There are four common themes, recognisable in the histories of many survivors of torture (Turner and Gorst-Unsworth, 1990; 1992). First, the survivor of torture has to face the intrusive thoughts, memories, dreams and flashbacks characteristic of incomplete emotional processing. The normal psychological mechanism by which the emotional content of everyday events is assimilated is overwhelmed by an extreme trauma. The scale of the emotional reaction is so great that the only viable psychological response to this distress appears to be an avoidance reaction. Both internal prompts and external cues continue to lead to recall of the torture, and this is associated with persistent avoidance of internal (for example, defensive emotional 'numbing') or external (for example, objects, people or places which resemble the traumatic experience) trauma-related stimuli. This condition has now been included in the American Diagnostic and Statistical Manual (DSM-IIIR; American Psychiatric Association, 1987) as a type of Post-Traumatic Stress Disorder (PTSD) and is a common sequel to many types of overwhelming trauma including natural disasters, war combat, and hijack survival.

Secondly, the survivor of torture often has to experience consequential losses. For people who stay inside the country of torture, these may include loss of status, money, home, occupation or even death of family or friends. For those who seek asylum in exile, these effects are often compounded by the additional losses of community, language, and culture. A process of 'cultural bereavement' (Eisenbruch, 1984a; 1984b) has been described. This may be potent in people who do not wish to leave their home country and whose affectional bonds remain firmly rooted there despite the enforced separation. Depression, either as a complaint or as a syndrome, is a common consequence of loss and appears to be particularly frequent in asylum seekers and refugees. For example, Mollica *et al.* (1987), in a study of South East Asian refugees living in America, found that major depression was the single most common psychiatric diagnosis, frequently co-existing with PTSD.

Thirdly, in a person who has experienced physical torture as a way of forcing a psychological change, it is hardly surprising to find that physical symptoms later come to have a variety of complex personal meanings and psychological significances. There are many examples of these mind–body interactive processes, well demonstrated in the chronic hyperventilation syndrome (Turner and Hough, 1991), but also seen in tension symptoms, sexual difficulties, and even in such apparently organic areas as memory and concentration.

Fourth in this list, probably most important of all, there is the effect on personal meanings and value systems. To survive in a world in which torture is not just a theoretical abstraction nor even merely a possibility demonstrated in the treatment of others, but in which it has become a terrifying reality for the individual survivor, almost inevitably leads to attitude change of some sort. For me, it will be to return to the struggle against oppression with even greater determination and commitment. For others, it will be a retreat into subdued acceptance or enforced exile. It seems to be in the nature of extreme violence that only extreme choices remain. Primo Levi (1987) described the same shift in priorities when, in the preface to his book *Moments of Reprieve*, he wrote that, for several years after writing and publishing his two early books, 'I had the feeling that I had performed a task, indeed the only task clearly defined for me. At Auschwitz, and on the long road returning home, I had seen and experienced things that appeared important not only for me, things that imperiously demanded to be told. And I had told them, I had testified.'

The therapist

Faced with the descriptions of torture earlier in this chapter and the even more tragic accounts which individuals may report in therapy, it is easy to feel overwhelmed by the size of the problem and to feel helplessly discouraged and deskilled. In part this may be an over-identification with the victim and is a response to the nature of their trauma. Mollica (1987) has written of the major feelings of hopelessness which at first were spread throughout his Indo–Chinese Psychiatry Clinic by 'the trauma stories' of the people being seen there. After all, these terrible stories have great power over the survivors and can come to have the same power over those who have to listen.

In working with survivors of torture, as in other clinical situations, it is important for the therapist to identify his or her own vulnerabilities as well as his or her strengths. The most dangerous action by the therapist is to allow his or her own emotional difficulties, unseen and unaware, to intrude into the therapy.

It is a common experience that those therapeutic skills which are used in day-to-day work in counselling, in medicine, in psychotherapy, are all useful in this work also. The initial feelings of discouragement and impotence are usually found to have been conjured from within the therapist; attempts to avoid a confrontation with the evil of torture.

One of the most contentious issues surrounding the therapist concerns ideological commitment. Where health and social workers are operating at great personal risk within a country of torture, they will usually be dealing only with one repressive regime and with its opponents. To be prepared to stand up for the rights of torture survivors in such circumstances requires considerable courage and may also be associated with a shared commitment for political change. For the survivor to be able to trust a therapist, and to reveal intimate secrets, this ideological commitment on the part of the therapist may need to be made explicit. On the other hand, in remote countries of asylum, it is more likely that individuals and groups will be working with survivors of torture from several regimes. An open commitment to a specific struggle or political group may hinder rather than help the development of a working alliance. However, it may be just as important to make a general human rights commitment. Workers from one European group have declared that, 'the commitment and the ideology of the therapist is a necessary precondition for a successful treatment outcome. It is an

absurdity to maintain a neutral attitude while listening to accounts of torture'
(Jensen and Agger, 1988).

Moreover, only if the therapist or group has developed some coherent
understanding of the social and political context in which they are working,
can they really start to address the ideological needs of their clients. It is
important that a client is not automatically reduced to passive patient status,
that both therapist and client are able to recognise that there may be parallel,
interacting understandings on a personal and psychological as well as on a
socio-political level. It should also be borne in mind that, for many survivors,
the therapist will be one of many people involved in the recovery process, that
ideological assistance is often also required.

The client

Survivors of torture are usually ordinary, healthy people. Some may have
been exceptional, for example, as political or religious leaders. Most had their
own strengths and disciplines to help them deal with torture and all
ultimately lived through the experience. Very few had need of contact with
psychiatric or counselling services before their assault. The common theme is
of an otherwise normal person, overwhelmed and damaged by unusual and
extreme trauma, yet in the end surviving it all. The survivor may be sad,
angry or hopeless, but often the lasting impression is of a quiet dignity and a
personal courage rarely seen in other settings.

All torture survivors are not the same, of course. Despite the similarities of
their experiences, there are not only personal but also cultural differences to
consider. In the Western world, the word 'torture' has consistently been
associated with the use of physical pain to force confession. The Cambodian
term, in contrast, is associated with the Buddhist concept of karma; survivors
feel they are somehow responsible for their suffering because of their karma
(Mollica, 1987).

These cultural factors can have profound significance. For example, an
Asian concept of self (interdependent, with a holistic psychosocial orientation) has been differentiated from the Western concept of self – as
independent, with an individualistic orientation – (Littlewood, 1990), and
several critical value conflicts between Indo–Chinese refugees and American
psychotherapists have been identified (Kinzie, 1985). Differences such as
these must be considered in the formulation of appropriate assistance.

The setting

There are certain organisational requirements which should be addressed
before considering therapeutic options. Foremost among these, there must

be a sense of safety and trust. Some refugee organisations only offer help to those who have already achieved asylum, believing that without the security this legal status carries, there is no possibility of meaningful work. This is to deny help to large numbers of people whose needs may be greater. It is a spurious argument, equivalent to denying medical aid to people solely because they are over a certain age and hence statistically nearer to death. Although psychological work with people who have not yet received asylum is often more difficult, it should be attempted and appropriate support should be offered. It has been argued that it is an important part of the ideological commitment to be able to demonstrate that help is available from the pre-asylum state onwards (Jensen and Agger, 1988).

It is also important to consider the safety of others. Parts of the history (for example, details of the escape route) may be sensitive. There is usually no need for a therapist to know details such as true names of people involved in the struggle or the escape. Simply to consider this issue and to be able to discuss this aspect of the history may be reassuring to the survivor.

The survivor of torture, probably more than anyone else, has a good reason to mistrust officials and official procedures. Anything remotely resembling interrogation must be avoided, but more than this it is particularly important to offer frequent explanations and opportunities for appropriate reassurance during history taking. Perhaps as a way of demonstrating independence from the therapist, it appears to be quite common for people to miss appointments or to arrive late. If physical investigations are indicated these must be explained with even more care than usual. The person who has survived electrical torture will see more meanings in the electrodes used in a routine cardiograph or electro-encephalograph than does the doctor who requested the investigation.

In many settings, it is necessary to work with interpreters, advocates or bi-cultural therapists. It is important to try and check that the survivor can trust a worker who may come from his own community. Bearing in mind the sensitivity of the information that the client has to relate, it may be necessary, at least at first, to accept a friend or relative as interpreter. This can cause problems, of course, and the session may become more complex with a need to consider the relationship between client and interpreter, or even the interpreter's own emotional reactions to the trauma. Others, chiefly those working with single country refugees, have helped to develop the role of the intercultural worker. However this language and cultural problem is resolved, the therapist should avoid using the interpreter only as a 'personal mouthpiece', a passive instrument of communication (Mollica, 1987).

Assessment and its dangers

The therapist will bring to the consultation whatever skills and techniques he or she already possesses. This can be valuable not just for the client but also for the therapist, by demonstrating that at least some of these skills have value. For a clinical psychiatrist, it can be reassuring to observe a beneficial effect of antidepressant medication both on depressive symptoms and on the intrusive features seen in PTSD. Similarly, it can be rewarding to see a rapid resolution of symptoms of hyperventilation syndrome once physiotherapy treatment is started. Indeed, in the latter case, as there are usually no active maintaining factors, treatment is often more successful than it is in normal hospital practice (Turner and Hough, 1991).

Yet there is a danger. For a person who has endured and survived, there may be a natural reluctance to see any of the psychological reactions in terms of medical illnesses at all. Rather, they are seen as evidence of a political process to which the individual had been subjected. 'Medicalisation' may be seen as a challenge to the ideological understanding of torture and may lead to a denial of the validity of any form of categorisation on the basis of symptoms. It is regrettable that these opposing forces so often lead to a destructive result. Just as a Cartesian dualism should be rejected in dealing with a psychosomatic complaint, so a similar dualism which opposes psychological and political understandings is equally meaningless.

The most satisfactory resolution to the questions raised by diagnosis is to apply an interactional model. Taylor (1979) has argued that it is always important to consider an interaction between three dimensions, the subjective symptom or complaint, the objective lesion or disease, and the socio-political context within which the person exists and operates. This applies equally to physical medicine as to psychiatry. For example, lung cancer caused by nicotine inhalation may have symptoms, has a recognisable lesion, and can only be fully understood within a society in which tobacco smoking is encouraged and pollution permitted. Similarly, the interacting subjective, pathological and ideological processes which operate following torture must each be identified and considered in an assessment of the whole person.

The therapy

An approach to the understanding and evaluation of appropriate therapy for survivors of torture and other forms of organised violence is still in its infancy. Nonetheless, some common themes emerge from the literature and are supported by personal experience. For example, the processing of emotionally charged memories is usually prevented, both by the high levels of distress they cause, and the avoidance reaction which inevitably follows. A therapeutic approach has to be able to deal with this distress in a different way. From the theoretical and clinical ideas of Horowitz (1976) and Rachman

(1980) on emotional processing, it seems that a gradual engaged exposure to these memories is likely to be most effective. Offering a survivor the opportunity to talk can be successful, particularly with flexibility in the timing of sessions. For some, long sessions of several hours may be required if they are to be able to approach the trauma without being overwhelmed (not dissimilar to critical incident debriefing after natural disaster). Brief recall with high levels of distress may serve to sensitise the person even more to the torture experience.

Mollica, in his writing, confirms that the 'trauma story' must be seen as the 'centrepiece of therapy' (Mollica, 1987). This may be a hidden secret (such as a rape trauma), which is nightly reviewed in the survivor's nightmares. However, telling the trauma story serves not just to assist in the processing of the emotions with which it is associated; it is also the first step in the construction of a new story, a new understanding of the past and a new hope for the future.

Testimony, initially used as a technique of political opposition to the human rights abuses in Chile, now provides the general basis for psychotherapy with survivors of torture and other forms of organised violence. By 'making previous life history – political commitment, personal relationships, work and social connection – meaningful in the present and in the future', it allows the survivor to reclaim a personal space and a sense of self worth. As Schlapobersky and Bamber (1988) describe it, this is a reclamation of personal time and space, a recovery from the consequences of torture to a lifespan which the process was intended to destroy.

The technique in its original form began with one or two interviews with a therapist; these were devoted to eliciting basic personal information including a first account of the political repression, and to establishing a therapeutic relationship. In subsequent sessions, the client would then be encouraged to tape-record a detailed description of the events leading to the present symptoms. The therapist's role was chiefly to clarify and expand this description by asking simple questions. The transcript of the testimony record was reviewed in therapy, the final product being a written document (15–120 pages) that had been edited jointly by client and therapist.

The therapeutic value of this procedure was reported by Cienfuegos and Monelli (1983), who found that anxiety and depression symptoms both remitted. Giving a testimony meant overcoming the pain of remembering, but more than this, it helped survivors to 'integrate the traumatic experiences into their lives by identifying its significance in the context of political and social events as well as the context of their personal history'. Aggression could be directed appropriately, and fragmented experiences could be restored to a wholeness within new personal and ideological understandings.

By allowing, indeed encouraging, a sense of personal dignity, it places the survivor within a treatment setting in which he or she is an active participant. Bearing in mind that torture affects ordinary people who have many personal strengths and resources, it is particularly appropriate that therapy should depend on self-help principles as much as possible. Although some have advocated a more prescriptive approach (for example, Somnier and Genefke, 1986), many would prefer to describe therapy as a process of active recovery rather than one of passive rehabilitation.

This technique, often modified to meet different needs (for example, Jensen and Agger, 1988; Lincoln 1988), has become established as one of the major therapeutic approaches. In summary, it has several beneficial aspects. First, the technique provides a good basis for gradual processing, keeping within the individual's limits of tolerance. Secondly, it may be used by some survivors as a legal document, a witness against torture and torturers. Thirdly, by describing in detail what really happened, each action is set in a context. The surrender under pain may be easier to accept; the political nature of the violence may be understood. It has been said that the purpose of torture is to make a political pain into a private personal pain; the aim of therapy is to reverse this by reframing the experience (Jensen and Agger (1988); Lincoln, 1988). Fourthly, it may help the survivor to understand and accept sometimes ambiguous feelings towards the torturer, working within the contrived, perverted intimacy of the torturer–victim relationship.

Naturally, any technique will have important limitations if applied to all survivors of torture, regardless of the presenting complaints; it is important to recognise and respect individual and cultural differences. There will often be multiple symptoms, including many somatic complaints: for example, a long-term painful impairment in walking from falaka, persistent headaches, abdominal discomfort, back pain, sleep disturbance with nightmares and insomnia, persistent sadness and pessimism, isolation, and difficulty in trusting others or forming close relationships. It is essential in approaching any of these that a whole person approach is adopted. Careful and detailed physical and psychological assessment, the avoidance of unnecessary physical investigation, the ability to offer appropriate reassurance and to understand some of the common interactive processes affecting mind and body, are all important.

Equally, it is important to consider the person within his or her own context. This means not only acknowledging the cultural background of the individual, but also recognising the importance of interpersonal relationships and the impact of enforced separation. Couple, family and community approaches may all be required (see Svendsen, 1987; Jaffa, 1992).

The extent of the cultural dislocation of exiled survivors has its first impact on the therapist when interpreters or advocates are needed in the assessment and treatment process. However, it has a much bigger and more immediate impact on the client as soon as they arrive in the new host country. The isolation of the asylum seeker, first from family and friends, and now from other people with barriers of language and culture, may be critical impediments to recovery. A therapist working with asylum seekers and refugees from many global conflicts, has to learn about aspects of many different cultures as well as the culture of violence itself in a world of repression.

Intercultural therapy may present challenges but it may also prove to be very satisfying. Of course, there are situations where language poses a real barrier. For example, a man from the Middle East with very limited English presented for therapy but he was only willing to visit his therapist alone, for fear that he would cry in front of another man from his own country. In this case, the early sessions were carried out with the aid of a dictionary. Yet the enforced use of the dictionary constrained both therapist and client to examine the cultural narrowness of language itself. Later the use of language education became a potent method of helping the client to regain self-confidence and move away from the entrapment of perpetual political conflict with others from his own country.

Finally, in this client group, intercultural group work has been used to advantage. One constraint in applying group work to refugees who have been tortured is that for many it is hard to have sufficient trust in someone else from the country of torture. It is common for refugee groups to have been penetrated by agents from the home government and information offered too freely may be abused. Paradoxically, a group containing people from many different cultural backgrounds and geographical areas may prove to be particularly powerful. The communication which can take place between people with such a common experience can transcend culture and even sometimes language (Schlapobersky and Bamber, 1988).

Secondary victimisation

A common reaction to trauma is to hold ambiguous views about perpetrator and victim. This is demonstrated very clearly following rape, when the victim may have to withstand accusations that she enticed, encouraged or in some other way was responsible for the man carrying out the sexual assault. Following torture, similar situations may be found both in relation to provision of services and also occasionally in the reactions of the therapist to the therapeutic relationship. These intrusions in countertransference need to be acknowledged and dealt with if they are not to risk greater harm to the client.

Conclusion

In this overview of therapeutic needs and possibilities, the problems confronting the survivor of torture and other forms of organised state violence have been set within a psychological, cultural, and ideological context. It is argued that each of these must be considered before approaching therapy. Testimony, a specific technique, has now been widely adapted for use in different contexts and serves many of these purposes. By setting the experiences of the individual firmly within a cultural and political context, it is possible to facilitate psychological recovery from symptoms as well as improved understanding of their social and political causes. It is also possible to help the survivor start to create a new life, to retell the trauma story, and to step forwards with dignity into a future that holds hope and opportunity.

Notes

(1)   In *submarino* torture, the victim's head is held under water, until water aspiration or unconsciousness occurs. The water is often contaminated with excrement.

(2)   In *falaka*, the victim's feet are beaten with a light cane or whip. This process is extremely painful and may be repeated frequently. Even years later, there may be soft tissue damage which causes pain on walking more than short distances.

Appendix

Case Examples for Teaching and Group Discussion

The following set of four teaching exercises were originally devised by the group working at Lynfield Mount Hospital for the 1983 Transcultural Psychiatry Society workshop in Bradford. They are based on actual consultation cases. Since then they have been extensively used and modified by the editors. Each case presents a problem of the sort that we might encounter in social work or clinical practice.

How to use these exercises
We have found these exercises most helpful in group discussions either as part of a course or for teaching seminars. Ideally, at least two hours are necessary to complete each one. It is a good idea if every participant has their own photocopied set of each case study used (copyright has been waived). The lecturer (or facilitator) should be familiar with the content of each study, and with the page of suggested procedure.

None of the exercises have a 'right' formulation or solution: they are to be used to discuss the relevance of medical versus social interventions; psychiatric diagnosis as opposed to psychosocial formulations; the relevance of racial attitudes to the origin of the problem and the interventions suggested; the role of culture, gender and class.

To what extent are the interventions suggested by members of the group acceptable within the client's cultural expectations? Elaine Arnold's example in this volume (Chapter 11) may serve as a guide here.

As an accompaniment to each case, we have suggested a few of the possible questions which might emerge. Other questions may be more relevant in different teaching contexts. Again, the point is to open up themes and to develop awareness of the issues (for example, the intervention proposed may not fit into the client's cultural expectations), not to achieve some sort of consensus on intervention. Do not avoid any feelings or processes which are developing in your group during the discussion: they are likely to mirror the actual clinical situation.

CASE STUDY A: ZOHRA BIBI

Suggested procedure

1. Read Sheet A (1) (A letter written by a consultant psychiatrist after visiting Zohra Bibi at home.)

Can we make a provisional diagnosis at this point? Should we?
Which points are selected out as of particular interest and why?
Any thoughts about the psychiatrist? Sympathetic? Useful?
Is the language Hindi?
What religion is Zohra? Does it matter?
Does the presence of the family make it easier (or more difficult) for the doctor to assess the problem?
Does it make any difference if the doctor is English or Punjabi in origin? Why?
What do we mean by 'Mrs Bibi'?
What should the medical team do next – if anything?

In fact they decided on early out-patient appointment.

2. Read Sheet A (2) (Psychiatrist's notes)

Do we learn anything new? 'In Pakistani'?
Was an out-patient appointment a good idea? Could she be psychiatrically ill? Why?
Do we pursue a 'medical', or a 'psychotherapeutic' approach? Why? Or both – why?

In this particular case, the team concerned had decided to use a social worker and find out more.

3. Participants can now choose any interview or available report. (Sheet A (3) – A (12), interviews with Zohra Bibi, her husband, her father-in-law, her mother-in-law, her brother-in-law, his wife; diagram of the family tree and glossary; housing report, employment report; economic report.

Possible questions:

What groupings of family members do we want to see again? Why?
Zohra seems to be able to speak English . . . comments?
Is it appropriate to identify Zohra as the patient? Are the interventions suggested consistent with power in the family?
Does Zohra need psychiatric treatment? Is she perhaps paranoid?
How 'British' are the family? All to the same degree?
Do the family dynamics include members in Pakistan?
Can we ignore the medical aspects given the focus on sickness?
Do family members all share the same explanatory model of what is going on?
What are the advantages and disadvantages of seeing Yasmin and Raffi?
Do professionals have anything to offer? Would the family be better off without any intervention?
Can we help individuals change without assaulting their own values and norms?

Can we work with the husband? The father-in-law? The mother-in-law?
Are family dynamics of any significance given the various reports on employment etc?
Is the problem 'cultural'? What does that mean?
What about the miscarriage? Should Zohra see another doctor?
Should Zohra and Khalid be encouraged to set up their own household? Why?
What are the advantages and disadvantages (and ethics) of psychologising this family's difficulties?

Is the family's culture felt to be at fault? Is it less adaptive in Britain? Why? Is a detailed knowledge of it necessary? Should they see the traditional doctor (hakim) now visiting London?

4. Group issues

How have the different ethnicities of participants in the group affected discussion? Has it raised any questions between group members which need to be addressed?

5. Conclusion

Any general thoughts about possible intervention in this case? Much of the discussion may have been about cultural differences, translation and knowledge of culture. How relevant has this been? Is racism in Britain also an issue? Does the case study offer a stereotypical British view of 'Asian families'? What is it?

CASE STUDY B: BEVERLEY CAESAR

Beverley Caesar is due to appear in court.

Suggested procedure

1. Read Sheet B (1) (The report by a probation officer at the request of the court.)

Any thoughts as to why we start with a probation report?
How does the presentation of the information for a court determine the way we see the problem when reading it? How does this reason affect Mrs Caesar's account?
Does Ms MacDonald believe the police or Beverley?
Any comments on Margaret MacDonald's language – 'factually similar', 'paradoxical', 'truculent', 'West Indian dialect'?

Beverley Caesar presents the issues in terms of 'race', the probation officer in terms of 'culture'. Are they mutually incompatible?

2. Read Sheet B (2) (Another court report.) How does this report differ?

3. Read Sheet B (3) (Report from Dr Wilson, Prison Medical Officer.)

The members of the group are likely to be very sympathetic to Beverley at this point! How common is her situation? Does it seem exaggerated (The letters here are, in fact, copies of actual ones.)

4. Read Sheets B (4) (Consultant psychiatrist court report) and B (5) (Another psychiatrist's report to Sylvester Chapal).

How helpful has the 'medicalisation' of the case been for Beverley?
Can she trust Margaret MacDonald? Could you?
Any thoughts on Dr Mason?
What will the court decide? What should the court decide?
How much have we learnt about Beverley from the different ways different people have seen her? What is her explanatory model?

In fact, to the surprise of many people, the court decided not to accept the recommendations of Drs Wilson and Morningside, but instead placed her on probation for two years, with a condition that she receives treatment from Dr Mason.

The terms of the Probation Order were explained in court to Beverley and her mother, and Beverley expressed willingness to comply with them.

Dr Mason stated that in-patient treatment was not necessary at the present time, but he would send an out-patient appointment in about a fortnight. Beverley left the court with her mother. Two of the youths also charged with assault in the same incident (who had previous records) were sent to prison, another was bound over, and one was acquitted.

5. Read Sheets B (6) and B (7) (Letters from and to Ms MacDonald.)

Ms MacDonald appears to be a thoughtful and conscientious person. She is aged 29, married, white, middle-class. Is she disqualified, as she fears, by her colour? (Or by her ignorance, prejudice or other characteristics revealed in the report?)
Would it be preferable to have a black probation officer?
What is the relative importance of colour, sex, age, skill and empathy in this situation?

What assumptions have members of the group been making about Dr Mason (MRCPsych)? Is he white or black?
How might the prospects for family therapy differ in each case?
What led members of the group to make assumptions about him?
Is family therapy appropriate? If so, who should be involved? Beverley? Gertrude? Paulette? Winston?
And what staff? Dr Mason? Ms McDonald? Someone different?

6. Group issues

How have the different ethnicities of participants in the group affected discussion? Has it raised any questions which need to be addressed before finishing?

7. Conclusion

Any general thoughts about culture versus race? Is 'culture' an issue? Whose culture? The Caesar family's? The white professionals'? Both?
Does the case offer a stereotyped perception of black families? If so, what is it?

CASE STUDY C: KATHLEEN WILKINSON

A case conference has been called by a clinical psychologist.

Suggested procedure

1. Read Sheet C (1) to Sheet C (7) – the request for a case conference, the later psychiatric referral to the psychologist, a social work report, a report by a community psychiatric nurse, the clinical psychologist's later report, a medical summary, a message from the psychologist after he organised the case conference. Any initial thoughts? What might be happening?

The case conference. Sheet C (8) (Kathleen's phone call) is available. So is Sheet C (9) (clinical case notes). Do they raise anything? How?

2. Inform the group that Kathleen is white/British.

Kathleen's ethnicity has never been specifically mentioned. How relevant is it? Have your group assumed the case will be of a black patient? Are they now disappointed? Is race only relevant to black and ethnic minority groups?
How does the ethnicity of the professionals affect their perceptions?
The psychologist was born and trained in the Irish Republic; the community psychiatric nurse was born in Trinidad; the social worker and the junior psychiatrist are British-born whites; the consultant psychiatrist was born in Calcutta and attended medical school in London where she trained in psychiatry.

What about 'culture'? What, if any, differences are there between the Wilkinsons' norms and the supposed 'British' norms, in, for example:

(a) being a good mother (or father)?
(b) being a good wife (or husband)?
(c) who handles the finances?
(d) tolerance levels towards delinquency, promiscuity, child abuse, poverty?
(e) attitudes to happiness, poverty, tax avoidance, madness, propriety?
(f) extent and style of 'inner-directedness' or its opposite?
(g) views on how one should present oneself to strangers?

What, if any, bias is shown by any of the professionals involved in the case and if so, is it due to the professionals':

(a) expectations from persons of the same sex (or opposite sex) to themselves?
(b) self-image of being in a 'helping profession'?
(c) own professional role?
(d) individual political or religious attitudes?
(e) own social class norms?

What, if anything, could be accomplished by a family session? If there is one:

(a) which members of the family should participate?

(b) which of the professions involved should participate in it?

(c) where should such a session take place, in the Wilkinsons' home? In an office at the hospital? In a social service office? Somewhere else?

3. Group issues

How have the different ethnicities of the participants in your study group affected the discussion? Has it raised any questions between group members which need to be addressed before finishing?

4. Conclusion

Does the case offer a stereotypical perception of the white working class? What is it? Or of women? Why?

CASE STUDY D: KATERINA ZBIGNIEWSKI

Suggested procedure

1. Read Sheets D (1–3) (Extracts from Katerina's medical notes) and Sheet D (4) (a letter from her son).
Does the interview with Maria (D (2)) make you question the impression from the previous day?

Dr Brown prescribed anti-psychotic medication (Sheets D (1–3)). Was this appropriate? Any other possibilities?

How might we describe the personalities of (a) Mrs Zbigniewski, (b) her late husband, (c) Maria, (d) Peter?
Any thoughts about the quality of the information we have so far?
What else do we need to know to help this family more effectively?
What do the group think about Mrs Zbigniewski's feelings about her black persecutors?

2. Read Sheet D (4) – Any thoughts?

It was felt appropriate that a Polish-speaking social worker would visit.

3. Read Sheet D (5)

Has the social worker learned anything which we could not have gained through using an interpreter?
This social worker is of Polish origin himself: what difference might this make? Any fresh thoughts about Maria's role?
How responsible does she feel herself?
Has any member of the group asked about the results of Mrs Zbigniewski's medication?

4. Read Sheet 6, a note made by a junior doctor in the hospital [KW is Dr Weinstein, the consultant who first saw her].
Does any member of the group suggest contacting the priest?

5. Pass out sheet 7 and discuss how relevant this information is to our understanding the situation. Does the group make increasingly fewer 'medical' suggestions as we gain more information?
Should we share this information with the family? How could it make a difference? Can the Church do anything to help?
Dr Weinstein's father was a Jew from Eastern Europe: any thoughts as to how he might feel himself?
Why has Paul only been mentioned now? Do we need a family tree? If so read sheet 8.
Are we doing everything that could reasonably be expected? Is the problem 'under control'? Any ideas as to what might happen next?
In fact nothing happened for a fortnight. Then. . . .

6. Hand out sheet D (9)!

At present we have in the hospital: Mrs Zbigniewski who has been brought to the psychiatric ward by the porter and has not yet been formally admitted to hospital; Maria Katzewicz in the out-patient department, in tears, being comforted by Mr Jakes and Dr Weinstein; Peter (Zbigniewski) Wilson and his wife and two children are waiting in the reception area.

The staff involved are the Consultant Psychiatrist, Dr Weinstein (who saw Mrs Z on 31.8.89 (Sheet D (1)) but not since, and has seen Maria on 1.9.89 (Sheet D (2)) and this morning (Sheet D (9)); the junior psychiatrist, Dr Dorset who saw Mrs Z and Maria in the out-patients on 21.9.89 (D (6)) and has had a preliminary look at Mrs Z this morning; the duty social worker Mrs Jones who has been asked to assess whether Mrs Z should be detained in hospital. The Polish social worker Mr Harek (D (5)) is not available today; the report he wrote after 12.9.89 has only just been typed and the hospital staff has not received it yet. Mrs Jones could go and obtain it if necessary.

7. If the group agree, read it (Sheet D (10)).

8. Before further discussion, read sheet D 11, and then return to D 10, the Polish social worker's second report.

Do we accept his assessment and recommendations unreservedly?

Do we learn anything new, directly or indirectly?

If the report had been received earlier, would different actions have been taken? In fact, only now do we learn about Mrs Zbigniewski's life and problems, and her feelings from Mrs Z herself. Up to now, everyone has been talking *about* her, not *with* her. Is this because of perceived language difficulties?

Is what we have been looking at 'a problem', not 'a person'? What do we do now?

9. Group issues

How have the different ethnicities of participants in your own group affected the discussion? Has it raised any questions between group members which need to be addressed before finishing (particularly Mrs Z's attitudes to her neighbours)?

10. Conclusion

What sorts of therapeutic intervention are most helpful? Is she too old, too Polish or too psychotic for psychotherapy? Any general thoughts about culture versus race? Is culture an issue? Whose culture – the Zbigniewski family's, or the professionals', or both? Mary/Maria? What effect might past political events have on the family and Dr Weinstein's attitudes to compulsory treatment? What cultural assumptions have been shown in the different reports? Does the case offer a stereotyped perception of Polish families? Or of women?

Case study A: (1)

Psychiatrist's letter to GP

RE: Zohra Bibi (aged about 23)

Seen at home at your request. Also present: husband (Khalid) and for part of the time mother-in-law and sister-in-law, plus one or two of the latter's children. The history was obtained from her husband, as others only speak Punjabi (or is it Hindi?). He speaks fluent English with a Yorkshire accent.

The main complaint is of many bodily symptoms developing over the past two years, especially since a miscarriage nine months ago. At first there were periods of intermittent headaches (frontal) with aches also around the back and shoulders and coldness in the hands and feet with generalised weakness. At such times she tended to retire to bed and be unable to do any housework.

For the past three months she has been a frequent visitor to the GP's surgery. He had recently referred her for investigation to Dr F (Consultant Physician) but no physical illness was detected. Mr Bibi complained that nobody had told them what the illness was, and pills from the GP (tranquillisers) gave only temporary relief. The husband felt they should also have done an X-ray of the head.

More recently she has been spending large amounts of time lying down refusing to talk to anyone and also often refusing food. She has also had a number of 'attacks' in which she is described as 'out of her senses'; she becomes restless, talks 'rubbish', complains of feeling hot, tries to rush out of the house and may become angry and abusive – on one occasion she even struck her mother-in-law. For a few days now she has stopped eating altogether with considerable weight loss. At nights she is often restless and noisy.

Past history: Mrs Bibi came to Britain about three years ago, soon after her arranged marriage, for which her husband had gone to Pakistan. He had been in Britain from an early age and all of his immediate family is here. They live in his parents' house which is also shared by his married brother, his wife and children.

According to her husband she was very well prior to this illness but he does not know of any medical history prior to her coming to this country.

On examination: She was lying on a couch with her back turned and hiding her face in her veil. Her replies mumbled and brief. She appeared apathetic and flat but was able to indicate the sites of her aches and pains. She said she did not eat because she wasn't hungry. She did indeed look thin, pale and unhappy. When asked how she felt about the loss of her first pregnancy her husband replied that it was the 'will of Allah' but it had certainly made her 'weak'. There was no evidence of obvious delusions or hallucinations.

The whole family were very concerned and anxious and pressed for her admission, but she shook her head and adamantly refused.

Case study A: (2)

Psychiatrist's notes

Three days later – notes of early out-patient attendance.

Patient accompanied by husband and father-in-law (Nur Mohammed, who was at work during the domiciliary visit).

No apparent improvement in her condition. They had discovered that food given to her had been thrown out of the window. She has been observed coming down at night and making some food for herself.

Patient again withdrawn and flat. When pressed she eventually said (through her husband) that her food was being poisoned and that was why she was ill. Husband thought that this was rubbish. He explained that 'she believes a lot in all that kind of superstitious stuff' – like 'magic'. He pointed to a leather amulet she was wearing round her neck – which she had got sent from Pakistan – and which she claimed was keeping her alive. He thought it was 'a lot of mumbo jumbo' and what she really needed was admission and some 'real medicine'.

Father-in-law, who has very poor English, gave a long speech mostly in Pakistani, in which he also emphasised how ill she was but he asked if we would let him take her to a famous doctor he knew in London for some special injection.

Asked about life at home her husband commented: 'We are a very close family', and appeared puzzled at the suggestion that her illness might relate to family tensions – 'We don't have any problems' – 'It's her health we are bothered about – she needs medical treatment to make her strong again then her troubles will go away'. Husband reluctantly translated that his wife had asked if we could help them get a house of their own – both he and his father dismissed this suggestion – following which they had a somewhat more animated discussion in which she also joined. Husband explained that it was 'nothing important'.

Case study A: (3)

Zohra's account

Hasn't the doctor come today? Why have you come instead of him? I'm ill, can't you see? There are too many people in this house, always bothering me, always asking me questions. Questions, questions, questions, you're driving me mad.

(After some time, and having finally cooled her down.) How do I feel? I'm still very weak, and I've got a bad headache. Those tablets they gave me at the hospital were quite good, they gave me some relief, but most of the pain has come back now, it hurts here – and here – and here. It's so bad I can hardly move.

Before I left Pakistan I was very healthy, it's only since I have been in England that I have grown so weak. At first I felt all right, but there was so much to do. This house is very big – I had never seen a house with so many storeys before, there are four from the kitchen to the attics. And so much work to do. So many rooms to clean. So many clothes to wash. So many mouths to feed. And my bhabhi with a young baby too.

When I was strong I could do all the work, but now I am so sick what can I do? I try to help when I can, but my sas gets very angry, and says I'm useless and lazy. When I'm as sick as this, how can I work?

I was really looking forward to coming to England, so many people from our village had come here, and ever since I was very small I had heard stories about it – how everyone had cars and television and dressed in fine clothes. And my husband's father is my mamu, so I thought I would really be treated well.

I was at first, but it didn't last long. I discovered later that my sas had wanted my husband married to somebody else, a cousin of Yasmin's and since Yasmin is her chacha's grand-daughter they were very close. In fact they never gave me a chance. My sas always favoured Yasmin, and made me do all the work.

But then it got worse and worse, they were plotting together. My mother got very concerned. After I lost my baby she sent me this tawiz. She got it from a very holy pir who lives in the mountains behind our village. I have to wear it round my neck all the time, to keep evil things away.

It worked quite well for a while, but then I think they must have found something stronger. I began to grow weaker and weaker, and look at me now. I'm only young, and I'm growing old very fast. England has turned out to be very bad. Even my husband is turning against me. He leaves me alone all the time with those two, while he goes off to clubs and places. England does very bad things to Pakistani boys. They forget about religion, and forget to respect their wives, and go with English prostitutes instead.

And I'm just left here at home, growing weaker and weaker. What can I do? Of course I try to be very careful, especially about my food. That's how they make me ill. That's why I threw out that food the other day, I could see they had put something in it. But even if I make my own food, I'm not sure it will make me any better, they will find other ways. Just living in this house makes me ill. You've got to help me. But what can I do? I can't go back to Pakistan. There would be too much shame. But I can't survive like this either. What can I do?

Case study A: (4)

Khalid's account

It's since we got to England that Zohra's health began to change. Perhaps the climate didn't suit her. She often got sick, so she even lost the child when she got pregnant. I don't know why that happened, but now she has got all sorts of silly ideas into her head about the way people are poisoning her. It's rubbish of course, she should have left all that kind of stuff behind her in Pakistan. But that's why she threw the food out of the window, you know, she thought it was poisoned. Everyone got right upset about that, especially my mum.

I don't know why it is, but mum has really turned against her. I know Zohra sometimes says bad things but she doesn't really mean it. It's only because she's sick. That's why she doesn't do her work either. She's not lazy, she's sick. We must find a doctor to cure her, though I'm not quite sure about this hakim my dad's got in mind. Perhaps she should have some more X-rays and a blood test, it's weakness in her bones, you know. Can you get her taken into hospital for treatment?

Unhappy? Why should she be unhappy? She always wanted to come to England. Of course she misses her mum, but she's bound to anyway. My sister often tells me how much she misses us, now she is married.

Lonely? No it can't be that. She has got lots of company here at home. Of course I'm out quite a lot, I can't stand the quarrelling that goes on half the time. But our women are like that. They keep each other company, and the lads get together separately. Pakistani families aren't like English families, you know.

Where do I go? All sorts of places with my mates. Where can you go when you're on the dole? We just hang about, and sometimes go down the club to play snooker.

Night club? Oh, have you been listening to all that rubbish from Zohra? She thinks all clubs are like the places you see in movies, so she's got this idea that we have dancing girls all over the pool tables every night! So she's started thinking that I'm going around with English girls, and might get infected and all that. Sometimes she just goes on and on about that, it makes me right fed up – especially when she gets the big freeze, and won't even talk to me. She only has to think about pool halls and she freezes up just like an iceberg. It's stupid really, when it is all in her imagination.

But I don't see what all this has got to do with it really. Zohra is ill and weak, that's what the trouble really is. If she was stronger all these family problems would go away. So why are you asking me all these questions? It's finding out what's wrong with her and getting her some medicine that really matters.

Case study A: (5)

Nur Mohammed's account

My home is near Chaksvari in District Mirpur, and I first came to Britain twenty five years ago. I worked in a foundry in Birmingham at first, and then came to Bradford. For the past eight years I have been working nights as a spinner, and so far, mashallah, I have not been made redundant.

For the first fifteen years I was by myself in England. My wife and children stayed in our village with my father and brothers. Those were hard years, because although I made three visits back home, the time between them was so long. Ten years ago I called my wife to join me, and then I could see my children every day.

I was happy at first to have my family all around me, but now I sometimes wonder what it is that I have been working for all these years. My house is troubled, and nothing seems to be at peace. My sons show me too little respect, and often quarrel with each other. Now the women have started too – many evenings I am glad to leave the house to go to work.

Living in England is really destroying our families, you know, and sometimes I wonder why I do all this work. All my life I have been working, and now at last I have some property. I have a fine new house just outside Chaksvari, some land, and a row of shops for rent. It belongs to us all, of course, not that my sons seem to bother about it. My sister's husband is looking after it all for me just now.

Of course my sister is also very worried about Zohra's illness, she often sends messages asking if she is well. I don't know what has happened to her since she has arrived in England – perhaps the cold weather doesn't suit her. I think we should all go back to Pakistan, we would be much healthier there.

But in the meantime some cure must be found for her. She is very sick now, and a woman who cannot work is bound to be in trouble. You know the doctors in the hospital – can't you persuade them to give her some really strong medicine to make her better. Sometimes, you know, they don't give our people the best medicine, just because we are not English.

That's why I was thinking of taking Zohra to a private doctor. My friend at the mill was telling me about a very clever doctor from Bombay who will be visiting soon – last time he was here he cured my friend's niece, who was suffering from the same kind of weakness. He charges two hundred pounds for a single treatment, which is very expensive but Zohra is my sister's daughter, you know, and her disease is causing so much trouble.

Case study A: (6)

Shaffia Bibi's account

You can never predict how a daughter-in-law will turn out, especially when you don't get a girl from within your own family. Some work, some don't. Some are respectful, some are shameless. Some are strong, some are weak. Some produce many sons, others produce none at all. Some bring honour to the family, others drain it all away. Much depends on the girl's own family, but you can never tell.

But if the choice is bad, what can you do? Can you expect respect where none has been taught? Can those who are weak be made strong? Can stones turn into pearls? For how long can anyone afford to keep a barren cow when a fresh young calf could take its place?

Of course, I do my best to treat my bahus well, I love them just like my own daughters. But we are growing very concerned about Zohra now. She behaves so strangely, and sometimes she says very bad things. How can she expect people to respect her when she says such things?

If she is ill she should be treated – we have spent a lot of money taking her to doctors. But what sort of disease is it? Will the rest of the family catch it? And now other people are beginning to talk about our family.

It is all making Khalid very unhappy. He's getting quite thin now, and his skin is going black. It's very bad for him. He deserves better than this: that wife of his is making him ill.

Case study A: (7)

Raffi's account

You shouldn't be surprised at all this, because women quarrel all the time in Pakistani families. It's in their nature. So there's my wife going on all the time about how she wants me to buy a new house; she doesn't have any idea how much it would all cost, especially when I'm just trying to get the business started.

An awful lot of trouble comes from silly quarrels, you know, like when Zohra arrived here my mum felt her dad should at least have helped out with the air ticket, but our dad said that was OK because she was so close to him anyway. You know she's his bhatiji? Anyway, my mum got right narked at that, and then started picking over all the things she's brought with her. She had a tough time really, except when dad got home.

But so did my wife too, when we first got married. It's nothing special. The trouble with my brother is that he's too soft, really. He should get that wife of his sorted out, but he just lets her get away with it. He listens to her too much, and then starts keeping away from me too. I used to be really close to Khalid before all this started, we had plans to go into business together. And now when I could really do with his help, he backs off.

It's breaking up the family, is all this, and it doesn't do any of us any good. If I were him, I'd give her a good thrashing.

Case study A: (8)

Yasmin's account

With three young babies to look after, how can I find the time to prepare everyone else's food? It's easy for those who have no children to lie down and be ill, but I can't do that. Whatever happens I have to feed my little ones.

Now that she is ill everyone expects me to look after the whole family as well as my own children. Even if I ask her to help me, she is always too tired or too ill. But now I'm having to be very careful. Three weeks ago Ghulam, my little one, fell ill – he was so bad we almost had to take him to hospital. So now I take great care to see that none of them eat anything from her hands. You can't be too careful.

Of course we heard so much about her from abbaji before she was married, and of course when she arrived here abbaji always used to favour her. But she has been here for a long time now; she can't expect to sit around like a guest for ever.

She thinks she's very educated, but does passing eighth class mean that women don't have to cook and to wash and to clean? Of course it's easy enough to lie down and make a lot of noise just to avoid your work, but is she really ill? If you ask me she is just lazy, and perhaps spoiled and jealous too. Nothing more than that.

Case study A.9

Family tree

Significant members of the household are related as:

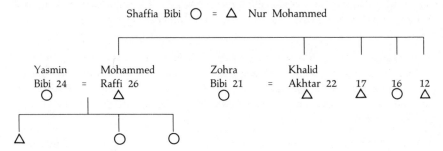

Glossary

abbaji	– father (also used by daughter-in-law for father-in-law)
bhabhi	– sister-in-law
mamu	– uncle (mother's brother)
sas	– mother-in-law
tawiz	– talisman; amulet
pir	– religious leader and healer
hakim	– doctor of Unani medicine
bhatiji	– niece
bahu	– daughter-in-law
nacha	– uncle (father's brother)
mashallah	– God willing
chacha	– father's younger brother

Case study A: (10)

Housing report

The Choudhry family live in a stone-built terrace, probably built around the turn of the century. Once this would have been a very respectable neighbourhood, but for years now the housing stock has been very ill-maintained, and is for the most part very run down.

The Choudhry's house is on the larger side, with three bedrooms on the first floor, and two large attics, recently extended through the construction of two dormer windows. Although the Choudhrys received an improvement grant, and all the necessary work was carried out, the house still looks run down. External paintwork and interior decoration are in very poor condition.

This is a joint family household, and their living conditions can definitely be regarded as seriously overcrowded. Two of Mr Choudhry's married children still live at home with their parents, and one couple has three further children of their own. In addition, two nephews of Mr Choudhry seem to be long-term visitors.

Since the house only contains seven living rooms, and the household a total of fourteen persons, conditions are clearly grossly overcrowded, but Mr Choudhry angrily rejected any suggestion that it was time his married sons moved out. A formal request for one or the other of the families to move would be necessary to gain sufficient priority for them to have a chance of being swiftly rehoused.

Case study A: (11)

Employment status

Nur Mohammed has worked as a spinner on permanent nights at Ball End Mills for the past ten years. Although there is a severe recession in the textile trade this company still seems to be in good shape, and the threat of closure which once hung over it now seems to have receded. With ten years' service behind him, Nur Mohammed is only likely to be made redundant if the mill closes.

Mohammed Raffi worked for the same company for two years, but was made redundant three years ago; soon afterwards he went into business as a market stall holder, selling cheap garments. After an initial struggle to get started he is now reasonably well established, but the recession is also having a significant effect on his business. Customers have less to spend, and large numbers of other Pakistanis are now trying to enter market trading. To compete, margins have to be cut to the bone, and profitability is very low.

For a while Khaled Akhtar thought he had done better than his brother. He worked in the carding room at Greensleeves Yarns, but the company suddenly ceased trading eighteen months ago. Khaled has had no luck in finding another job, and says that it is now too difficult to do as his brother has done and go into market trading. Since he was made redundant he has spent a great deal of time playing pool.

Case study A: (12)

Economic resources

Nur Mohammed owns outright the house in which the family live, and has almost finished paying off the loan he obtained to convert the attic. He is also part-way through building a new house for himself in Chaksvari, but progress came to a halt because of a disagreement with his brothers over some additional farmland which they chose to purchase. Nur Mohammed managed to sort these difficulties out during his recent visit to Pakistan. Nur Mohammed also has £2000 out on loan to his younger brother's daughter's husband who lives in Walsall.

Nur Mohammed also provided some of the basic capital which Mohammed Raffi used to start his business. The rest came from Raffi's own savings and his redundancy money. Otherwise Raffi took goods on credit from Pakistani suppliers. Raffi now has a two-year-old Volkswagen van, and a stock that he reckons is worth at least £5000. But he is trying to put every possible scrap of capital into the business.

Khaled Akhtar's only income is Supplementary Benefit, much of which he spends in the pool hall.

Case study B: (1)

Castlebridge Magistrates Court

Beverley Caesar, 14B Corinthian Terrace, Grantly.
d.o.b. 13.6.1973

Charges: (1) Theft
           (2) Resisting arrest
           (3) Assault

Adjourned hearing on 25.8.90

Social Enquiry Report by Ms M J MacDonald, Senior Probation Officer.

I interviewed the accused and her mother Mrs Gertrude Caesar at their home on 22.8.90. I further interviewed her mother on 21.9.90.

Circumstances of the offence

The account given by the accused is factually similar to the Police depositions but Beverley's interpretation is different and she pleads not guilty. According to her she was leaving Lutterworth's store where she had bought nothing, and was stopped by a security guard who accused her of stealing a dress. She had a dress in her bag, which she had bought earlier in the day at a different shop. She claims that if she had been given an opportunity to do so she would have produced the receipt, but instead she was arrested and the contents of her bag, including the receipt, were impounded by the Police. She admits to losing her temper and hitting the Police Officer, but claims that the four youths who appeared on the scene and are also charged with assault on the Police were unknown to her previously. She stated vehemently that she believed the police would not have proceeded against her had she been white, and she is of the opinion that police officers attempt to provoke black persons into losing their temper so that they have an excuse to arrest them.

Background

Beverley Caesar is aged 17 and was born in the Frixpeth district of Grantly. She lives with her mother Mrs Gertrude Caesar who came to Britain from Jamaica two years before Beverley's birth. Soon after that her relationship with her husband became strained and he left. Mrs Caesar had four children by her first husband, and has had three others by two different men since her marriage broke up.

Mrs Caesar is a stout, motherly woman who seems to be devoted to her children. She was at pains to point out that she had given all her family 'a good Christian upbringing'. She seems most concerned about Beverley's welfare, and says that she does not understand what is happening to young people in Britain, and that they all seem to have 'gone crazy'. She is particularly concerned because Beverley recently got mixed up with 'bad people', including her current boyfriend, Winston, who she described as a 'no-good Rastaman'.

Because of this she stated that Beverley was beyond her control and that she needed firm discipline. In fact she seemed quite pleased with the prospect of Beverley being removed from her current associations to a place where she might be taught to behave better.

Mrs Caesar drew comparisons between Beverley's behaviour and that of her eldest daughter Paulette. She regards Paulette as 'a credit to the family' because she is in regular employment as a bank clerk, and is always smartly dressed. She proudly showed me photographs taken at the christening of Paulette's second child – which seems to have been a rather paradoxical event because Paulette is not married. However Mrs Caesar's main hope seems to be that Beverley might be persuaded to behave more in the way that Paulette does.

Interview with Beverley

I found her truculent and suspicious, convinced that no justice could be obtained from white people, and regarding herself as being a victim of racial victimisation. She also seemed to think that I was in league with her mother against her. Her behaviour was very casual. She dresses in a careless fashion, her hair unkempt, and she was very resistant to thinking about her future. My efforts to gain her confidence were not very successful on this initial meeting. Whenever we came close to discussing anything significant she tended to switch into a form of West Indian dialect which I was unable to follow.

Beverley's behaviour is clearly somewhat disturbed, in the same manner as that which I have seen in quite a number of West Indian families. It could well be that this is partly because there is no strong father figure in the family.

As the court is aware, Beverley failed to attend the adjourned hearing on 25.8.90 and she also failed to keep the appointment made for her to see a psychiatrist on 14.8.90. She was therefore arrested and detained in Wigley Remand Centre from 30.8.90 to the present. I understand that reports from Wigley will be available to the court.

I visited Mrs Caesar again on 21.9.90, and this time she gave a somewhat different account. She has changed her mind about Beverley's 'wickedness' and now claims that she is basically a good girl who has been wrongly accused. She now seems to think that she is fully capable herself of dealing with any problems which Beverley may have.

Recommendation

Beverley is handicapped by adverse home circumstances, and has also developed unnecessarily hostile attitudes to those who are seeking to help her. Nevertheless, I would respectfully suggest that she be made the subject of a probation order, provided that she expresses willingness to co-operate with a probation officer.

(Ms) M MacDonald
Senior Probation Officer

Case study B: (2)

Report from Miss K St J Beale, Headmistress, Grantly High School

I was obliged to exclude Beverley Caesar from this school in November 1988 due to her increasingly disruptive behaviour. Although not lacking intelligence she had over the last year or so gone out of her way to argue with her teachers, and had systematically disregarded school rules with respect to dress. Despite the fact that I and my staff made considerable efforts to talk through her problems (hers is a single parent family) she has persistently chosen to reject our advice. Since she also goes around with a small group of other children of similar background, who were causing so much disruption in an otherwise happy multi-racial school, we decided that we had no alternative but to exclude them.

I fear that Beverley will continue to get into trouble until she abandons her single-minded campaign to break every rule which she encounters. I do hope some means can be found to persuade her to cease to behave so anti-socially, and that she will soon begin to realise that those who behave in such a manner can only do themselves harm.

K St J Beale, BA
Headmistress
Grantly High School

Case study B: (3)

Wigley Remand Centre, Wigley, Lincs.

Beverley Caesar   Admitted for assessment for one month 30.8.1990
                      Due at Castlebridge Magistrates Court 27.9.1990
                      Offences   (1) Theft. (2) Resisting arrest. (3) Assault on Police
                             Officer.

The accused had been remanded on bail on 5.8.1990 for psychiatric and Social Enquiry Reports, but had failed to attend for psychiatric examination and had failed to attend court for the adjourned hearing on 25.8.1990. Remand in custody was for the purpose of psychiatric observation. She was admitted to the hospital wing but her behaviour proved too disruptive and it was necessary to transfer her to one of the main wings.

Report

During her stay here Beverley has been consistently truculent and unco-operative. Much of this behaviour may be attributable to the effects of a broken home and incorrect handling in childhood, but there is also evidence of an insidiously developing mental illness, i.e. paranoid schizophrenia. (See also report from Dr Morningside.)

When asked about the offences with which she is charged Beverley has persistently protested her innocence, and any disagreement with her version of events quickly provokes rage and unreasonable accusations against the questioner and all 'white' persons, whom she appears to regard as her persecutors. This paranoia is not susceptible to reasoned discussion and has the features of a primary delusion.

At times her conversation becomes fragmented, garbled and incomprehensible, including neologisms and mispronunciations of common words. She frequently refers to some kind of biblical fantasy involving conquering lions, days of retribution and 'the walls of Babylon falling down'. Further enquiries about what she means elicit only withering scorn.

Her behaviour is unpredictable and attention seeking. She insists that she is a vegetarian 'because of her religion' but absolutely refuses to discuss what that is (see above). She constantly protests that the clothes she has been given to wear are dirty, even when they have been washed. She appears obsessed with cleanliness, and has a bath at every available opportunity. All staff have noted her constant aggressiveness and say that she 'has a chip on her shoulder'. At times she has been destructive of clothing, tearing off a strip of cloth with which to cover her hair, and this appears to be compulsive behaviour, possibly in response to hallucinatory instructions.

One of the staff here who is also West Indian suggested that some of Beverley's statements were similar to those made by members of the Rastafarian cult, but this seems an insufficient explanation for her disruptive and delinquent behaviour because:

(a) Beverley was born and brought up in Britain and has never lived in the West Indies.

(b) I am told that her mother is a convinced Christian and Beverley was brought up as a Christian.

(c) Her paranoia and unpredictable changes of mood and behaviour do not have any logical or reasoned basis and seem to be completely impulsive.

(d) She does not have 'dreadlocks'.

Opinion and recommendation

In my view this girl is seriously emotionally disturbed and requires further assessment and treatment as an in-patient in a psychiatric unit and should be detained under Section 60 of the Mental Health Act.

PT Wilson, MB, BS
Senior Medical Officer

Case study B: (4)

Valley View Hospital
Castlebridge

The Clerk
Castlebridge Magistrates Court

Dear Sir,

Beverley Caesar (aged 17) 14b Corinthian Terrace, Grantly
Currently at: Wigley Remand Centre.

At your request I arranged to see the above-named in my clinic on 14.8.90 in connection with charges of theft and assault. She failed to attend, and I subsequently went to see her at Wigley Remand Centre, Lincs., on 13.9.90.

I regret to say that my visit (which occasioned me no little inconvenience to arrange) was almost entirely fruitless, since Ms Caesar was totally unco-operative and proper psychiatric examination was impossible in the face of her intransigence.

Nonetheless, having discussed her case with Dr Wilson (PMO) and members of his staff, my observations support the impression which they have gained, namely, that she is suffering from a combination of personality disorder (aggressive psychopathic variety) and incipient or actual paranoid schizophrenia. The evidence of this is in her aggressive, unco-operative attitude, refusal to discuss her symptoms even when it is obviously in her own interests to do so, and her fixed belief that she is a victim of persistent persecution by an organisation which she refers to as 'Babylon'. She exhibits manneristic behaviour and there is some evidence that she experiences auditory hallucinations.

I consider that she is in urgent need of psychiatric treatment in hospital and because of her lack of insight and unreliability it will be necessary to arrange her detention in the first instance in secure accommodation. I regret that I have no such accommodation available at this hospital and suggest that application be made to the Regional Secure Unit at Grimsleigh Hospital.

A note of my fee is enclosed.

Yours sincerely,

J. Crossley Morningside FRCP, FRCPsych, DPsy
Consultant Psychiatrist

Case study B: (5)

Dr JP Mason, BSc, MRC Psych
Consultant Psychiatrist

6, Cardigan Villas
Cardigan Park
Grantly

23.9.90

Sylvester Chapal LIB
Rights Officer
Grantly CRC
79C, Roodly Road
Grantly

Dear Sylvester,

As requested, I went across to Wigley to see your friend Beverley Caesar this week. She was pretty unco-operative, but eventually opened up a bit. There's no doubt the girl's rather unstable at present, and she's got in with a fairly anti-social crowd, but I can't find any evidence of schizophrenia or anything which needs hospital treatment. Certainly there's no cause for a Section, and that must be resisted.

I don't know what the evidence is that she did or did not pinch the dress – she still says it was planted, but I have my doubts. Anyway, you can play that one whichever way you think best, but my guess is we might get probation with luck.

I enclose a formal report saying the usual things which you can hand up to the bench. If you want me in court please let me know in good time and I'll come (but remember, some of them down there don't like my face all that much, after the Doreen Brown case).

Best of luck,

Joe

Case study B: (6)

Casterbridge Probation and After-care Service

Bishops House
Grantly

30.9.90

Dr JP Mason BSc, MRCPsych.
Consultant Psychiatrist
High Park Hospital
Roodly

Dear Dr Mason,

Beverley Caesar

As you know, the above-named appeared at Castlebridge Magistrates Court on 27.9.90 and was convicted of theft of a dress. The other charges against her were dropped. She was placed on a probation for two years with a condition that she receive psychiatric treatment from you. I shall be assuming responsibility for her in the first instance.

I understand from your secretary that an appointment has been made for you to see her on October 10th at 11.00 am.

May I make two suggestions? First, I would like to come with her on that occasion. (I am not absolutely sure she would get there unaccompanied, despite her promises.) Second, do you think it would be helpful if Mrs Caesar came along as well? Beverley is living with her mother and although they seem to be supportive to each other at present I suspect that family tensions play some part in Beverley's problems, and perhaps we should be thinking in terms of family therapy?

There is a further problem which bothers me. Because I am myself white, Beverley may find it difficult to trust me, so would it be better to try to find an Afro–Caribbean Probation Officer to take over? The only one likely to be available is much older, but I am not sure if this matters.

Can we discuss, preferably beforehand, how to proceed when we meet on October 10th?

Yours sincerely

Ms Margaret MacDonald
Senior Probation Officer

Case study B: (7)

Ms M MacDonald
Senior Probation Officer
Grantly

Dear Ms MacDonald,

I am writing to alert you to the fact that we have been very concerned to discover that two children, on whom we have been keeping an eye, Erskine Caesar aged 9 months, and his brother Darren, aged 2 and a half, are being looked after for most of the day by Beverley Caesar, aged 17, whom I understand you are supervising under a probation order.

The children's mother, Paulette Caesar, aged 21, is a single parent. Mrs Lovell, a health visitor attached to Roodley Clinic, has been visiting her regularly, but was extremely disturbed to discover that Paulette has just taken a full-time job, and left the task of childcare to her younger sister. I do not know how much substance there is in it, but Mrs Lovell tells me she understands that Paulette has a history of severe mental instability.

Mrs Lovell feels that there is a strong case for the children to be taken into care, but I feel that we should not take such a step without checking out the family a little further. I would be very glad if you could contact me as soon as possible about this.

Yours sincerely,

Gill Jacobson
Social Worker

Case study C: (1)

Case conference, 5th October, 1989

From: Patrick S L O'Halloran, Senior Clinical Psychologist
To: 1. Dr Biswas, Consultant Psychiatrist
        2. Mr Bill Ferguson, Senior Social Worker
        3. Sister Elizabeth Lister, Community Psychiatric Nurse

Re: Mrs Kathleen Wilkinson, 27 Cyprus Avenue, Salisbury Estate

I have just had yet another crisis phone call from Mrs Wilkinson. It seems to me that we are not handling this case right but I am not sure what the next step ought to be. I have had a word with the Consultant Psychiatrist and we decided to call a case conference between the four of us, as one way or another we have all been involved with Mrs Wilkinson since her last admission. Would 11 am next Monday, 10th October, be suitable for all of you? Please contact me.

To recapitulate: Kathleen Wilkinson has been on our books for nearly three years and has had three admissions over the past 18 months. She is 39 years old. Married, with five children: Michael 22, Tracey 18, Gary 17, Susan 15, and Kelly 4. The three youngest still live at home. The family live on Mr Albert Wilkinson's invalidity allowance. Kathleen's mother is still alive. She lives locally and keeps in touch as do Kathleen's two married sisters: Shirley c. 46 and Jackie c. 33.

I have been seeing her since May, at first on a weekly basis, lately about once a fortnight. It would be telling a lie to say that she is making no progress but she is playing some sort of a game which is frustrating to me and sabotages her own improvement. She seems to improve her behaviour for a bit, reaches a point where she appears at my office with make-up and beautifully dressed, reports that all is well, and wonders if she should 'waste my time' by coming again. Misses an appointment or two; then suddenly I get a crisis phone call, begging for an immediate appointment. This has now happened at least four times. I gather that her attendance at the clinic is also pretty erratic.

The latest crisis seems to be an objectively serious one. Her eldest son Michael (the one with the long criminal record) has just succeeded in involving the whole family in trouble with the Law through some stolen goods.

I enclose copies of our letters and memos to each other concerning Kathleen. Dr Sweetman is sending you a summary of the case notes.

Case study C: (2)

Psychiatrist's referral to clinical psychologist, February, 1989

From Dr Biswas to Mr O'Halloran, re Kathleen Wilkinson

I would be grateful if you could have a look at this lady with a view to supportive psychotherapy after her discharge.

She has taken three overdoses within one year: the last time it was touch and go. She was still suicidal afterwards whilst at the infirmary. Within 24 hours of admission here, however, she seemed to improve and by the time I saw her she said she 'didn't know what got into' her, she did not know why she did it and can she now go home, please? I explained that this was impossible; she wept a little but complied. Compliance and lack of resistance to anything and anyone is her most characteristic trait. The woman has no stuffing in her, in addition to being uneducated and inarticulate. Having seen the husband, I am not particularly surprised at Mrs Wilkinson's spiritlessness. He is an aggressive, overbearing, truculent, rigid, selfish man. Incapable of realising that his wife is seriously ill, he is merely aggrieved that her hospitalisation interferes with his own comforts. He is off work with a 'bad back' and is at home all day yet still expects his wife to do everything. They live on his social security. They obviously live on the breadline; Mrs Wilkinson says they can 'manage all right' with money. (I have now asked for a Social Report on the family.)

Mrs Wilkinson is not psychiatrically ill, she is merely an inadequate personality who cannot cope with the economic and interpersonal stresses brought about by her husband's loss of employment. Her overdose, however, was a serious one and we cannot discharge her without some safeguards. Seeing you would be one of these.

I would hope that regular sessions with you could help in future to make her feel most supported and to defuse any future crisis that is likely to make her suicidal.

Case study C: (3)

Social work report

From Mr Ferguson to Dr Biswas, re Kathleen Wilkinson

The Wilkinson family consist of Mr and Mrs Wilkinson and their three children: Gary 17, Susan 15 and Kelly 4. There are two older children who have now left home. The Wilkinsons' sole income is the husband's Social Security. They live on the Salisbury Estate in a pre-war three-bedroom semi-detached Council house. The fabric of the house is in very bad condition (rotting window frames, leaking drains, rising damp, etc.) but so far the Wilkinsons' repeated requests to the Council for urgent repairs have had no effect. Theirs is definitely a case for re-housing but Mr Wilkinson refused to give me permission to take steps in the matter, saying that he would like to discuss it with his wife first, after her discharge. Until I raised the matter, the idea of re-housing never seems to have occurred to them.

Mr Wilkinson was born in South Africa but lived in Britain after his parents returned here. He is aware of the hopelessness of their economic situation. He is a skilled machinist but has been out of work for years. By now he has begun to show all the signs of suffering from the reduced quality of life due to unemployment. The house is very shabbily furnished, everything is old and worn and of poor quality, except for the brand new video system which seems to be his only escape from grim reality. He says that it has been bought outright with money won on the football pools. His only hobby had been photography but now he can't afford it.

My unannounced visit found the house very clean and surprisingly tidy; obviously a lot of trouble was being taken to keep it so. Mr Wilkinson said that his wife was very houseproud and that he was working very hard to keep everything up to her standard. At the same time he complained bitterly about his wife's female relatives who, he said, interfered in everything, 'butting in all the time'. I did not like to question his word but it seemed to me that the impressive cleanliness of the house may have been due more to these ladies' efforts than to his. Their help was probably essential for running the household, whether Mrs Wilkinson were in or out of hospital. Luckily, Mrs Wilkinson's mother (Mrs Nancy Sugden) does not live too far away, one of the sisters (Mrs Jackie Crowley) has a car and the other (Mrs Shirley Bonnison) lives along the same bus route as the Wilkinsons.

The relatives' continued involvement seems to be necessary for the sake of the children as well. The little girl (Kelly) is sickly; she has an ear infection, wets the bed, etc.; seems to be taken to the doctor all the time. The older girl, Susan, has been in some trouble for glue-sniffing and for school avoidance. The son, Gary, has recently had a warning from the police for joy-riding in a 'borrowed' vehicle and without a licence. It is obvious that Mrs Wilkinson is an inadequate mother who cannot discipline the children. Over the last few years Mr Wilkinson has become too apathetic to function as a father. This has become more marked since Mrs Wilkinson's first psychiatric illness. Apparently she has increasingly become more inconsistent, unpredictable, unreliable, and often suicidal, in addition to her usual 'softness', panicking and other inadequacies. In these circumstances it is not surprising that Mr Wilkinson sees no choice except to opt out.

In view of the children's problems and the housing situation I think that it may be a good idea if we were to keep an eye on the Wilkinsons even after Mrs Wilkinson's discharge from hospital.

Case study C: (4)

The Community Psychiatric Nurse's impressions, April, 1989

From Sister Jackson to Dr Biswas, re Kathleen Wilkinson

(You asked me to write down the things I have been telling you about the Wilkinsons, so here they are, but kindly note that this is not a proper report.)

I have been visiting Mrs Wilkinson twice a week since her discharge ten days ago to give her her medication because it has been decided that it was not safe to let her have too many tablets at once.

She is fine at the moment, coping, cheerful, not suicidal at all. I have always thought that she is not the one who should be under the psychiatrist but the husband. Not much of a man, Albert Wilkinson. Never mixes, just stays in all the time, no friends, never had any. He has to be right every time though, lays down the law of the land at the drop of a hat. Carries on wonderfully about the rights and wrongs of the working class but it was Kathleen who had to put up with having all the children. He is beginning to feel his age though and at least he does not bother her much nowadays so less chance of another pregnancy, though I would not reckon it an impossibility as some people do not know how to age decently. Kathleen is a good wife. When Albert was still in work she would have the meal on the table as soon as he walked in through the door; she looks after him still. Keeps a nice home and she will not stand any nonsense from the children. She also puts up with her mother who comes and nags at her all the time though I cannot fathom how Kathleen can stand it. Kathleen is worth ten times the old woman, Mrs Sugden, Nancy they call her (she used to be quite a girl or so I have heard). Kathleen's sisters are not much better; Kathleen is the only respectable one. And Kathleen is a worker. She has always gone out to work, evening cleaning, when Albert was still at the mill, now any job she can get hold of, cleaning, packing, serving behind a bar, anything. All in addition to looking after her home and her family. She is a good mother too. Pity she has been so unfortunate with her children, though of course living at Salisbury has had a lot to do with it; it is the worst Council Estate in town; thieving, mugging, vandalism, break-ins, you name it, it happens at Salisbury. Michael, Kathleen's eldest, has always been in trouble, but he has recently moved in with some woman so at least whenever the police come for him it is not to Kathleen's that they come. The eldest daughter is now away too, at college, that must be a relief too; Tracey used to be a right handful. Gary is fast following in Michael's footsteps, Susie sniffs glue and Kelly is shaping up to be a worse problem than her mother: asthma, bed-wetting, eating problems, not to mention a chronic ear infection that does not respond to antibiotics.

I believe that Kathleen's psychotropic medication is not the only thing to watch but somebody ought also to make sure she does not get rid of the coil or if she does, get some other form of protection; another pregnancy would be the end.

Case study C: (5)

Clinical Psychologist's first interview with patient

From Mr O'Halloran to Dr Biswas, re Kathleen Wilkinson

Although I had made Mrs Wilkinson's acquaintance when she was still on the ward, I did not recognise her at all when today for the first time she came to see me by appointment. She was dressed very well, looking smart and sophisticated.

Her behaviour, however, belied her appearance. She seemed tongue-tied and even when she uttered I had the greatest difficulty in understanding her broad dialect. She became more forthcoming and more comprehensible as the interview wore on, but there remained a certain amount of reserve, not to say hostility. (Perhaps she does not like Irish men: she may have done better with one of my colleagues.)

She is a controlling woman who had trained her family to leave all decisions and all responsibilities to her. It became impossible to continue this regime after the husband became redundant and stayed at home all the time; she found it increasingly hard to keep her hand on the reins but was reluctant to relinquish any of her power. She is also a devout Catholic and has not yet come to terms with the abortion she had two years ago. Unfortunately she dares not discuss her grief and guilt at home because the rest of the family are either non-Catholics or lapsed Catholics and they do not enter into her feelings but respond by saying that she is 'crackers'. She has particular difficulties with her mother who seems to be a confusing person, inclined to give contradictory messages and expects total loyalty from Mrs Wilkinson. Mother and daughter have a very bad relationship and the mother's presence has a detrimental effect on Mrs Wilkinson's marriage. Indeed Mrs Wilkinson, her mother and her sisters seem to run everything, shouldering Mr Wilkinson out of the way. There are communication difficulties between husband and wife at all levels.

She insists that all her overdoses were definite attempts to kill herself and had not aimed at controlling or blackmailing other people. This is hard to believe from such a person; besides, so many repeats of the same behaviour point to some function. At this stage, however, I cannot yet see what the function of the suicidal behaviour may be.

I have discussed anxiety control with her and have tried to relax her but she did not respond very well this time, though I hope that this will change. In addition to training her to relax I am planning also a programme to improve her communication skills and, later on, to give her marital therapy (always supposing that the husband is willing to participate in it). I shall be seeing her on a weekly basis for the time being.

Case study C: (6)

Summary of the case notes on Kathleen Wilkinson (October, 1989) by Dr Sweetman, SHO

Dr Biswas asked me to summarise the case notes for the forthcoming case conference but as there are a lot of inconsistencies in them, it was difficult to write a sensible summary.

Mrs Wilkinson was first referred in December 1986 by her GP and seen in OP by Dr Waterhouse early in 1987 on two occasions. She OD in February 1988. Admitted to ward 7 under Dr Waterhouse; discharged within the week. Attended one follow-up appt, then DNA. Another OD in June 1988. Admitted to ward 7 under Dr Billings. Discharged end of August 1988. Kept 3 or 4 OP appts, then DNA. Yet another OD in February 1989. Admitted to ward 7 under Dr Biswas. Discharged in April with safeguards involving community nurses, social worker, psychologists and OP appts with the consultant herself.

Over the years she has been treated by 3 different Consultant Psychiatrists, in addition to at least 2 Registrars and more than 4 SHOs.

She has been described as having difficulties in coping (by Dr Waterhouse) and as being inadequate and inarticulate with a poor self-image (by most doctors). In the opinion of nurses she 'carried on' with the male patients on the ward, a nuisance, a problem personality unable to get on with other people. Kathleen's sister said last year that Kathleen had been no trouble as a child, a model wife and mother, got on well with everyone; this year she said that Kathleen was a 'snob' who just could not take being poor. The sister seems to be in the habit of coming to K's aid in a crisis, e.g. she accompanied her on her first visit to the hospital in January 1987. Her husband was said to be 'very concerned' about her early in 1988 (note by Dr Waterhouse), 'depressed' according to Dr Billings later that year, but 'aggressive and self-centred' according to Dr Biswas in 1989.

At present Mrs W is:
(1) being seen in OP by Dr Biswas, nominally at 6/52 but she misses every other appt;
(2) being visited by Sister Jackson 1/52 with medication in small doses;
(3) being visited by Mr Ferguson on an occasional basis (last visit 6th Sept); and
(4) she sees Mr O'Halloran about 2/52 or so. Medication: Prothiaden 25 mg tds; Ativan 1 mg tds.

Fuller excerpts from case notes are available if anyone wishes to see them.

Case study C: (7)

Message about Kathleen's conversation, 6th October, 1989

From Mr O'Halloran

On Wednesday I rang Kathleen to tell her of our intention to have a Case Conference on her. Today she turned up without an appointment, just to deliver the transcript of a conversation she has had with a friend in August: 'To help you and the other doctors understand me better' but she apologised for it being 'a bit silly'.

The transcript (made from an accidental recording of a conversation) has some unusual features. One of them is Kathleen's surprising interest in politics; I did not expect her to feel so strongly about anything outside her immediate family, nor to have a grasp of such things. Another surprise is her preoccupation with contraceptives; this comes as news to me, she did not seem to be interested in discussing this sort of thing. Her general attitude to sex as shown by the transcript is also rather different from the way she usually presents herself. There is an unfinished sentence somewhere in the middle about 'not being fair to Albert' which is very puzzling. Perhaps I am letting my imagination run wild, but does she by any chance mean that the aborted child was not her husband's? This could be true if she is as bored with her husband as the first part suggests. Reading the transcript I was somewhat disturbed by the casual way Mrs Wilkinson shrugs off her younger son's delinquencies. I have also found her view of us a little disconcerting.

I could get you photocopies of the whole transcript if you are interested.

Case study C: (8)

Transcript of Kathleen's conversation with a friend (August, 1989)

[Note: Mondays and Wednesdays Kathleen takes her four-year-old daughter Kelly to the Salisbury Estate Playgroup. On a day in August she found a new Mum there who turned out to be an old friend of hers, Mrs Janet G. This woman had left the area some twenty years ago and has only recently returned: this was news to Kathleen and the two women had a long conversation. It chanced that this happened during a period when a research team was researching this playgroup in depth and, with the permission of the mothers, they taped everything that went on there for some days. Kathleen had more or less forgotten about it until reminded of it the other day by one of the playgroup leaders. Kathleen then asked if she could get a transcript of her conversation with this Janet. She says that the main reason why she wanted it was that afterwards she had fallen out with Janet and wondered just how many damaging things she has said about herself while letting her hair down. It was only later that it had occurred to her that the material may also be useful for therapeutic purposes. PSL OH]

'. . . Yes, I'm still married to Albert though there are times I'm not sure why. Well, you know what he is like. No, he hasn't changed, not much, not in all these years. I suppose I'm fairly fond of him, he is me kids' Dad after all and he up with our Mike in spite of everything, and give him his dues he means well. But, well . . . it gets you down, you know, at times, when you hear the same thing over and over again, day in, day out. "Let's see what the old boy has to offer", he says, every blessed day when he switches on the blessed telly. I could scream, I could, you know. Yes, of course, I tell him, told him last night and not for the first time either, I said for godsake say somewhat else once in a while. What? Oh, he just looked surprised like, and a bit hurt, he said "Don't be daft, Kathleen, you do carry on, don't you?" What? Yes, sure, business as before, never stopped to think I could have meant it, he said it again as soon as I turned away. I tell you some days I could just scream. In love, rubbish, what's that mean anyway? This new feller of yours must put some notions in your head, honest, Janet. I tell you I'm fond of him and why not I say. But being in love, oh dear.

Tell you what though, at least he's always good for a proper argument. Mind, he never opens a book, not him, gets all his facts from the old box. When he has any facts that is, mostly he'd rather argue without facts, much more in his line; thinks he's so clever. What about? Oh, politics, of course, he's always been old-fashioned Labour; and at times about religion though not so much now. I used to hold by the Pope and that, but I'm not so sure about it now, it's this here Polish Pope; too political if you ask me; he should stop gallivanting all over the world and find out about contraception instead. I mean how women cope with fifteen kids, them that are fool enough not to get the Pill I mean.

No, I'm not on the Pill, not anymore, it's me blood pressure, they said sorry, nothing doing, give me the coil. Bloody awful, I tell you. No, I'm not swearing, bloody is the word, the floods I get, oh dear, I wish they'd take it all out and have done away with all that. Mind you, at least now it don't hurt no more, I mean that there coil. The first one they gave me, it were terrible, I was in agony all the time, no I'm not joking, for months it gone on, they said I'd get used to it but of course I didn't I could have told them. Made me wait two whole months then they had a look and of course it's been put in all wrong, I were lucky it didn't kill me outright. No, they had said but you should have seen their faces. Half Family Planning came in to have a look. Yes, of course, at me privates, what else? Mind you I expect they thought I wouldn't notice or something, all very earnest. At last they took it out; that were just terrible, I passed out though, so maybe it could have been worse. Yes, I know I never fainted before but there's got to be a first time for everything. And then I were in such a mess they said I got to wait a bit before they tried it again; come back in another two months, only I wouldn't. Didn't want to go next or nigh that place ever again, just kept away. Only when I gone and got caught, didn't I, so I were in a spot, what with our Kelly that were not yet four, and Albert on the dole and that and besides, the whole thing weren't fair on him.

Why? Oh I don't know. I get all muddled and that and thought I'd best put a stop to it all, only they brought me round. Yes, I took some stuff. Oh, just some Paracetamol and some nerve tablets Albert had from the doctor's. What? Well, yes, being off work gets him down a bit, of course; don't know what to do with hisself all day, not much of a handyman he never was and gets ever so moody, though it's not so bad in the summertime, he can get the chance to potter outside, thank god, get out of me hair. But I tell you straight I dread the winter, it gets so you daren't open your mouth. Not much chance of him getting a job, not now, he's on the sick now, it's his back. Well, when I were so low he thought he'd best get a job, just some job, anything, and he were taken on at Hatton's, just packing you know but there were a lot of heavy lifting and in next to no time he gone and busted his back. He's on the sick now, a bit more money of course but no chance of ever getting work, not unless that there Tony Benn gets them to see reason, but that too has gone for a — though why you should be a Tory I'll never know and don't give the stuff about your Dad who knew Lloyd George or do I mean Disraeli? Alright, alright, I know there's no point talking politics with you, you are like most women, just bleating what some feller's drummed into them. Nobody to talk to, that's me trouble. Yes, there's always Albert, but it gets monotonous, I know by heart what he had to say. Most times anyway. And the women round here talk nothing but bargains and did I know that the police have been to the Turners?

Mind you, three cheers for them Turners, keeping the fuzz busy, at least then they're not after our Gary for a change. No, of course nothing serious, just gets bored, no work, nothing with a bit of security, been on one of them Yop things, but not much joy once it's over: no chance of anything else and they say "you've had the privilege, let someone else have a go now"; it makes you sick. The kids, they're a worry and no mistake but you can't keep them on a lead and it's not like when we was young, they expect to dress and go to discos and that. Of course it cost the earth, it cost all we have but we can manage alright and time to worry about a new suite once the kids have grown up, if we live to see the day.

Maybe we won't or I won't I should say, I'm not sure I want to. Live that long I mean. Specially when me Mam gets started on me, like this morning, I could've screamed, she came round just as we was setting out to come here. Always choosing the right moment to butt in, me Mam is, and it's never any use saying no. This time she fetched me some awful scarf, a present for you she says; it were a bargain. If it were; but it's best not to ask where she got it from. Turned out she come 'cos she wanted some pickle, surprise, surprise, our Jackie must have told her I been pickling onions, me Mam never could be bothered to take trouble over her cooking let alone preserving. So of course I mean she's not getting any younger and that, and she is me Mam after all. Yes, alright, there's no need to remind me, maybe she give me a hard time when I were younger, I know, I know, but that's all in the past now. No I haven't forgot it, not exactly.

I think on it only when I get right low, you know. Everything looks right black and hopeless and I start studying and then I remember all that as well, among other things, everything that's best forgot, all that's happened over this past twenty years and more. . . . Oh dear, I wish you hadn't got me started on this, I wanted to keep cheerful. I wish you hadn't made me cry, I got to see the doctor in a couple of hours, she'll think I've gone back to square one.

Oh, the nerve doctor, a Asian lady doctor but she is a lady too, posh I mean, ever so ladylike. Don't understand half of what she has to say but she means well I'm sure. Dead funny at times I must say. There she is in that there smart suit from Fraser's. I seen it in the sales, reduced to 110, no, not from, to, reduced from 200-odd and wearing shoes to match I should think and holds forth on the dreadful economic hardships of women, I ask you. All very well intended of course and it's intelligent conversation for a change but at times it's the other one. The other one is the psychologist doctor, an Irish feller but serious as anything. Yes, I have to see him once a week; it passes the time I daresay but when am I to get on with the work? I got a backlog of ironing as long as me arm. I'm supposed to be doing the ironing Tuesdays but Tuesdays now I go see this here Paddy, Mr O'Halloran I should say, and it takes the whole afternoon, what with getting ready and waiting for a bus and that, so the ironing gets put off. No, he don't talk a great deal really but goes on about me sex life, no, I don't mean it that way, don't be silly, years younger than me, I'm an old bag to him. Besides he wants me to take Albert along to see him but of course I don't, I'd never hear the last of it, and anyway who wants to stir things? And he thinks, this O'Halloran does, that I've been too soft with our Mike and he could be right at that. Our Mike, he's been in and out of trouble since he were that high and me hair's gone grey with worry. But now he took up with that there Linda Watson, Lilly Woods' niece, you may recall her, he's gone to live with her. No, they aren't married and if you want to go and do aught about it you are welcome far as I'm concerned, you won't get anywhere though; them two they'll just be as ignorant to you as they been to me, go on, why don't you give it a try? But honest, you think we haven't tried, me and Albert not to mention me Mam and Albert's father and our Shirley and even our Jackie too though how she could, it's a wonder. They just laughed in her face of course. Our

Shirley? Oh well our Shirley is quite another cup of tea as you well know. You'd best go and see her for yourself. Yes, they still live there.

Me in love with the doctor? I tell you she's a woman! Oh, the other one, no, of course not. Me with a smartie-pants Irish know-all with a college degree?! You must be joking or you must think I'm a worse case from what I am. No, he says me trouble is that I'm too bossy; that I should let Albert look after the bills and that. Only he don't ask what would happen if I were fool enough to let Albert manage the money. That's a laugh that is, anyway it's no job for a man. I have to pay the electric and the gas and the rent too, got to pay them meself even when I'm sick in hospital, otherwise we'd be cut off.

Yes, of course it's the fruit an' nut hospital, what else? I'm past caring, I'm getting used to it. They call me a head case, so what? Albert and me Mam of course and even the kids have started too, only I give them a crack when I hear them say it. I daresay the neighbours know too, you can't keep quiet that sort of thing, not on that estate and what with the ambulance and that. Once or twice only, maybe three times in all. No, of course, I'm not unhappy, what daft questions you ask, what would I be unhappy about? I had to go into the nerve hospital because I done it a few times. Took some stuff I mean, nerve tablets, only more than what I were supposed to. I can't now, there's a nurse coming Mondays and Thursdays, give me only so much at a time, so as I can't take too many all at once. Actually, I could if I wanted to, there's ways and means, only I don't want to, not no more, but it keeps them happy, watching me tablets I mean and Albert don't carry on so much about it neither. She is quite a decent woman, that there nurse, though talk about nosey! All them nurses and health visitors, they always want to see the dust and the toilet and the kitchen and do I air the sheets, I don't of course, who would, but I always say yes, it keeps them happy. But this one, she wants to know all, what's wrong with Albert's back, how's our Kelly, has our Sue gone to school and why do I let our Gary get mixed up with them West Indian lads. I'd like to see her try and stop him, how can you, when we live on that rotten estate and the Turner's Jim the same age as our Gary, they've been mates all their lives. But I don't mind her so much, the Welfare man is much worse, social worker he calls himself, the sort that think women are just cattle but goes on about social conscience. No, of course he don't come about the kids, how dare you?! I never been in trouble over me kids, I'm not one of them that get their kids taken off of them! Well, if you choose to take it that way. . . .'

Case study C: (9)

Patient's name:	WILKINSON, Kathleen: number: 86/1014

December 1986   Wrist-cutting episode. GP Dr Bar refers her to Dr T.C. Waterhouse, Consultant Psychiatrist.)

January 1987   Seen in OP by TCW. Came to the hospital accompanied by her sister who had to do some of the talking for her. At interview Mrs W was weepy, inarticulate, looked unkempt, wrist bandaged. She has discovered unwanted pregnancy, youngest child merely four years old, not intended further children. Husband on dole. 'Mild depression and anxiety due to an unwanted pregnancy in an inadequate personality. She has difficulty in coping, cannot control her children: husband on Social Security. Recommend termination of pregnancy.'

March 1987   Seen in OP by TCW. Tremendous change: came alone, well dressed, hair done, make-up, full of life. Came to thank TCW for arranging termination, said she was physically still weak but relieved. Reluctant to accept a further appointment.

April 1987   DNA further appointments.

February 1988   Overdose. Seen in infirmary by SHO Dr Khan: 'Says she meant to die, no point in living. Low self-image, inadequate, inarticulate. Clinically depressed'.

February 1988   Admitted on Ward 7 under TCW. Sudden improvement after admission. TCW saw husband: 'A pleasant, intelligent man, very concerned about his wife. Promised to help Kathleen more in the house'.

February 1988   Discharged within a week of admission. Rx: Mianserin 60 mg o.n.; Diazepam 5 mg t.d.s.

March 1988   Seen in OP for first follow-up appointment by Registrar Dr Cooke. Looking well, thanking doctors for help. DNA further appointments.

June 1988   OD. Seen in Infirmary by SHO Dr Palfrey: 'Says she does not want to live. Inarticulate, inadequate. Clinically depressed.'

June 1988   Admitted on Ward 7 under Dr P.S. Billings, Locum Consultant Psychiatrist. Sudden improvement after admission. Decision not to discharge her too soon in view of past history. PSB saw husband. Husb. insists he does his best to help his wife 'but it's no use' (?). 'He seems depressed too'.

July 1988   PSB saw Kathleen's sister: 'Says she cannot understand what has got into Kathleen: as a child she was the one who was no trouble, later model wife and mother, got on well with everyone, never any problems. The sister is an odd woman, actressy and large; restless eyes.'

August 1988   Discharged on demand from nursing staff: 'She is getting too used to hospital and getting in everyone's way. Carrying on with the male patients. She is a nuisance. There is nothing wrong with her, only a personality problem, cannot get on with other people.' Rx: Prothiaden 50 mg t.d.s.; Lorazepam 1 mg t.d.s.

September 1988   Seen in OP for first follow-up appointment by Registrar, Dr Verma. Grateful and well-dressed; 'all is fine', she says.

Oct–Nov 1988   DNA appointments.

December 1988   Attended with Dr Verma. Apology for missed appointments but says all is well.

January 1989   DNA next appointment.

February 1989   OD. Seen in Infirmary by SHO Dr Jones: 'Still suicidal, confused, inarticulate. Says she intends to die as soon as she is free.'

February 1989   Admitted on Ward 7 under Dr Biswas, Consultant Psychiatrist. Sudden improvement after admission. Dr Biswas interviewed husband; 'Aggressive and truculent, quite incapable of under-standing that his wife is seriously ill. A rigid, self-centred man, thinks he owns his wife. Less concerned with her than with his own comfort. Insists loudly that he is willing and eager to help: "I will do anything you say doctor" and says that he misses Kathleen. Then it turns out that he misses her mainly because he is "not much of a hand at cooking". His idea of help seems to be to visit her every day in order to moan at her, mainly about his health. They live on his invalidity; unfit for work for over a year with a "bad back" and thinks he is entitled to all the sympathy going. Youngest child aged 3 is ill with ear infection: Mr W sees this as added suffering for himself. The marriage has been going for 20 years.' Dr Biswas saw Kathleen; 'Pathetic, downtrodden, inarticulate. Says she now does not want to kill herself, she does not know what has got into her the other day, "everything just got to be too much", no particular reason. "I am real sorry doctor, you have all been so kind" and "I would like to go home now, please doctor, I won't do it again." Direct questioning elicited a "he is all right". I told her she cannot go home yet: she wept a little but put up no real resistance, obviously too browbeaten to argue with anyone. Asked about finances, she said they "can manage all right" which seems unlikely. (Get social report: perhaps the new SW could do it?) – No psychiatric illness; inadequate personality. Take her off all medication for the time being.'

February 1989	Referral to clinical psychologist by Dr Biswas [see Document 3]
Feb–March 1989	Discussions all round, to decide under what conditions she can be discharged eventually.
March 1989	Social report from Bill Ferguson [see Document 3]
March 1989	VRC interviewed Kathleen's sister: 'She insisted on seeing me. A sharp, tense and intense, wiry lady. She is convinced that "Kath is only putting it on, wanting sympathy. Has been a snob all her life. She cannot take being poor, there is nothing else wrong with her". Further questioning brought forth nothing tangible, merely "I just thought you should know, doctor". (Why all the spite?)'
April 1989	Discharged, on following conditions: 1. Follow-up in OP by Dr Biswas; 2. Medication at home twice weekly by Community Nurse; 3. Refer to psychologist; 4. Social Worker to visit occasionally. Rx: Prothiaden 25 mg t.d.s.; Lorazepam 1 mg t.d.s.
April 1989	Impressions of Community Nurse [see Document 4]
May 1989	First interview with clinical psychologist [see Document 5]
April–Oct 1989	Intermittent attendance at Dr Biswas OP Clinic.

Glossary

OP   – out-patients' department at the hospital
DNA – did not attend
SHo – junior psychiatrist (Senior House Officer)
OD   – overdose of drugs
t.d.s. – medical abbreviation for three times per day

Cast study D: (1)

Katarina Zbigniewski

Date of birth   27.10.1919   Roman Catholic/Widow/Polish born

31.8.89   Seen by consultant (KRW) on domiciliary visit at request of her general practitioner.

Presenting complaint: believes that she is being persecuted by her neighbours who she says want to get her out of the house so they can take it over. Shouting abuse in the street. Refused to let social worker enter house, shouted at her through the letter box. (Psychiatrist gained entry by visiting when the daughter (who lives with her) was at home).

History of present illness: (obtained partly from patient who speaks adequate English – but mainly from daughter). About six months ago the daughter noticed her mother was increasingly reluctant to go out of the house, started locking herself in when left alone. Husband died 18 months ago. Daughter (Mrs Katewicz) is a school-teacher (?widow), and they live together. Three months ago the neighbours started making extensive alterations to their house, patient disturbed by constant banging, builders rubble in back yard. Told daughter that she was being spied on. There is a mosque across the street, and patient claimed that she was being observed from there by men with telescopes and short-wave radios. Now thinks neighbours have made door through wall on first floor and 'hordes of Asian men' come through, wander about house at night. (NB the social worker is black.) For last two months has slept downstairs in armchair. Last week Electoral Register form delivered through letter box, patient became very disturbed, tore it up. Now thinks house being watched by police.

P.H. Impossible to persuade her to talk about her previous life at this time.

On examination: very agitated, spoke in mixture of English and Polish. Initially suspicious but later seemed to regard doctor as an ally, freely expressed paranoid ideas about the neighbours, mosque, police, etc: no insight. Broke off in middle of interview to shout angrily up the stairs in Polish (?at supposed intruders). Refused to take doctor upstairs to see alleged entry. ?Hallucinated. ?Thought disorder ?Mood depressed (appropriate?).

Refused to contemplate admission to hospital.

Provisional diagnostic formulation: paranoid psychosis? Early dementing process?

Treatment: Obviously necessary to have a further talk with the daughter in private. Appointment made for her to come to hospital the following day. No immediate urgency about treatment.

Case study D: (2)

1.9.89. Notes by K.R.W.

History obtained from Mrs Zbigniewski's daughter, Maria Katewicz, seen on her own.

Mrs Zbigniewski was born in 1919 in a village in eastern Poland, the youngest of a family of seven, most of whom were killed during the war. In 1940 she was taken to a labour camp in Germany where she had a pretty bad time. She used not to talk about this, but has referred to it once or twice recently. In 1945 she came to England and worked in a textile mill.

Married 1946, husband ex-Polish officer, and they settled in Bradford. He died 18 months ago with cancer.

Children (1) Maria born 1946, married aged 19 to a Mr Katewicz, a dentist, but divorced after 3 years and has lived at home ever since: qualified as a teacher after her divorce. (2) Peter, born 1952. (Maria thinks there was a miscarriage in between); Married 1976 (English wife) two daughters aged four and one; lives in Leeds, visits every few weeks.

According to Maria, mother was always a competent and hard-working person, with no psychiatric symptoms until recently. Has had a 'very hard life'. Used to speak English quite well but now insists on speaking Polish in the house. Attends church two or three times a week (Catholic) but now refuses to go unless someone, e.g. Maria, goes with her.

Maria thought at first that mother's illness was due to loneliness following death of husband, but now thinks that she is 'going senile'. Has become very dependent on Maria, watches at the window for her return from school, makes a fuss when Maria wants to go out in the evening. Until the last six months she never complained about the neighbours, but has always 'kept herself to herself'. It is true the building work next door did cause noise and mess, but 'no more than you'd expect'. Very houseproud.

Early life and family: Little known. About five years ago patient received a letter from an elder brother in Poland, thought to be one of the few remaining relatives. Spasmodic correspondence since but patient has difficulty in writing in Polish. (Can't write English at all.) Since recent political changes in Poland, started talking about returning there to live with this brother. Unlikely.

Family psychiatric history: Patient's son, Peter, saw a psychiatrist aged about 18 because he 'had got into bad company and drugs' but now 'seems to have settled down'.

Provisional diagnosis: Paranoid psychosis. Exclude an organic illness.

Treatment: There seems no way of persuading Mrs Zbigniewski to come into hospital. Medication (Stelazine 5 mg. t.d.s.) to be provided by GP, Mary will try to persuade her mother to take it. Polish-speaking social worker to visit. OP appt. to be sent in 2/52.

Case study D: (3)

5.9.89. (KRW) Telephone conversation with patient's GP, Dr Brown

Salient bit of information: He has known this family for more than ten years. The husband died of carcinoma of the prostrate and was severely ill for the last six months, indwelling catheter, etc. Wife and daughter nursed him devotedly. Maria is an 'absolute saint'. Mrs Zbigniewski rather limited in intelligence but both women are 'the salt of the earth'. No previous evidence of paranoia or instability in mother, it was the men in that family who were always the problem. Father was a drinker and gambler (though not an alcoholic) and the son followed in his footsteps as a teenager, financially irresponsible. (? drug involvement at one time ?) Now seems to have settled, good job in insurance, but does not do much for the family. Ought to give Maria more support.

Patient has longstanding mild high blood pressure (140/100), not on any treatment. When present symptoms started he examined her carefully and found nothing else.

Dr Brown will prescribe her tablets.

Glossary

OPD   – the out-patients' department at the hospital
3/52   – the medical abbreviation for three weeks
Registrar – a junior psychiatrist

Cast study D: (4)

Letter from Peter Zbigniewski

122 Buckingham Mount
Leeds 6

4.9.89

Dear Doctor,

I am writing to you about my mother who is your mental patient. My sister says she has gone funny since our father died but I don't think this is the reason because she was quite OK for about a year and in any case she is better off without him. She won't tell you this, but he was a drunkard and he used to give her Hell. He made our lives a misery when we were young especially my mother and sister because he bullied them. He made my sister get married when she was only young to Mr Katewicz who was also a right bastard, just because his father had been a friend of his. The best thing Maria ever did was to divorce him, but our parents never forgave her for it. I don't know how Maria has put up with it all these years. I had to get out and make a life for myself. They never accepted my wife although she has always tried to be friendly, my mother wouldn't even speak to her at the funeral. She always wants me to go and visit her but I don't take Jean and the children because there's always an atmosphere. Last time I went she blew up because I told her I was thinking of changing my name. I want to change the whole family to Wilson which is my wife's name because our little girl will be starting school soon and I don't want them to have the same problems I had being jeered at by other kids because of a funny name. My dad always wanted us to be Polish, he even made us learn Polish on Saturdays and go to church, though he never went himself.

I don't know what's wrong with mother but I think it's the neighbours that have upset her and weaken her head. That used to be a nice area but it's changed so much you might as well be in Pakistan. That's not racist, it's not their fault, but it's true. They just treat women differently, especially when they are alone. I don't think she'll ever get used to it, and it isn't fair on Maria having to stop in with her all the time, she needs looking after properly, she ought to go into a home. I hope you will be able to arrange that, it will be best for everyone. I know there are some very good ones.

Thank you

Mr Peter Wilson (Zbigniewski)

Case study D: (5)

Social History and Report Sheet

> Surname (Block Letters)
> ZBIGNIEWSKI
> First Names
> KATARINA
>
> 14 Springs Terrace
> Bfd 2

I visited the family on 12.9.89 but Mrs Zbigniewski was not at home, apparently one of her Polish friends had come to take her to church. Her daughter Mrs Maria Katewicz told me that since she started taking the medication two weeks ago she has been somewhat improved, and is less angry and aggressive though still has paranoid ideas.

I took the opportunity to talk to Maria. She is a good-looking, self-possessed woman in her early forties, who teaches biology at Foxton Middle School. Seemed calm and competent but expressed great concern about her mother, saying she did not know what to do for the best.

In view of the information provided by her brother I asked about the parents' marriage, and she eventually admitted that her father had been a heavy social drinker, spending most evenings at the WM Club, and he had a bad temper. Nonetheless she seemed to remember him with affection and said that she does not blame him for having made a life for himself outside the home because Mrs Zbigniewski was not very stimulating company. When I tried to explore this, she said that her mother had little or no education and no interests apart from her home and family. I asked Maria whether they had reason to feel persecuted by their neighbours and she said that she personally always got on very well with them. She teaches a lot of Pakistani children in school and likes them.

About her brother, Peter, Maria was defensive, saying that he had 'the right to make his own life'. She thinks he was always their mother's favourite and still is, but after his last visit the patient had been very upset. She has since learned that Peter is thinking of changing his name, and supposes this must have been the cause. The following day she asked Maria to write a letter for her to her Uncle Kazik in Poland, saying that she wanted to go back there to live with him. She wrote the letter at her mother's dictation, but thought it was silly: there has been no reply.

I gave Maria an opportunity to talk about her own marriage and divorce, but she declined, saying only that it was a good job she was free and available to look after her mother. This was said with a smile but she then left the room hurriedly, and returned after a few minutes with fresh make up; she apparently does not wish to do so.

I arranged to visit again next week to see Mrs Zbigniewski herself.

K. Harek
Senior Social Worker

Case study D: (6)

21.9.89. This lady arrived in OPD this afternoon. She was brought by her daughter and a priest: they were late because pt. had refused to come until the priest went and persuaded her. Dr Weinstein had left so I saw her as I was duty doctor. I have not seen her before and she does understand English. Mrs Katewicz says she is a bit better. She does not seem very disturbed but I think she is depressed. She had made them promise she would not be kept in hospital. They seem to be coping. Continue same medication and keep appt. to see KW in 3/52.

RKD (Registrar)

PS: Before he left the RC Priest said he would like to talk to Dr Weinstein about this family: advised to phone.

PPS: Suitable for medical student exams (with interpreter of course). Good 'cultural case'. I think she might come. KWW to arrange?

Case study D: (7)

23.9.89   Father Janovitch (Polish RC Church) phoned to request interview again. Talked on phone.

Wants to know how he/his congregation can help Mrs Z or Mrs K. After hesitation and much reassurance on confidentiality, etc., produced a bit of information, viz. Mr Z when alive always claimed to have been an officer in Polish Army: but he (Fr. J) 'happened to know this was untrue. In fact Mr Z was in Britain as a POW having been fighting in German Army (? reluctantly) and captured in 1945. He had been interrogated closely by British Officers for possible involvement in something nasty concerning the local civilian population in Eastern Poland. He successfully concealed this fact from his family and the Polish community (but Fr. J thinks Maria may have discovered the truth since his death). Fr. J. thinks this explains Mr Z's moroseness and drinking – 'he was living a lie all his life. Thinks it would be kinder for the family to remain in ignorance now, in particular, 'Paul . . . would hate his grandfather's memory'. This was the first time anyone mentioned Paul, I was surprised to learn that there is a grandson. Apparently Paul is the son of Maria Katzewicz, now aged about 22. Lived at home until 2 years ago. Described as intelligent and likeable boy. In teens became very patriotic for Poland, read books, asked questions ++, Polish flag on bedroom wall, etc., was planning to visit but prevented then by current political situation. 2 yrs ago joined Brit. Army, stationed in ? Aldershot.

KWW

Case study D: (8) Family tree

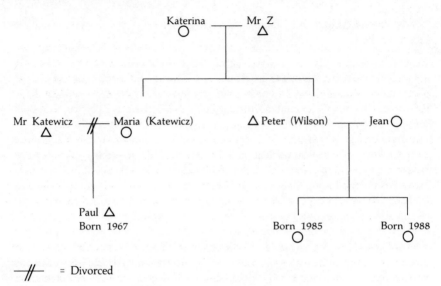

Katerina ——— Mr Z

Mr Katewicz —#— Maria (Katewicz)   △ Peter (Wilson) ——— Jean ○

Paul △
Born 1967

Born 1985   Born 1988

—#—   = Divorced

Case study D: (9)

Note by Psych. Registrar

8.10.89 9.30 am received telephone call from a Dr Appleby, a police surgeon. Mrs Zbigniewski taken into custody last night, after fight in the street, on Section 136. Apparently created a disturbance outside local mosque and tried to gain admission. There was a swastika chalked on the door and it was first thought that Mrs Z had done this but police later caught white youths doing same thing elsewhere and think it was done before Mrs Z arrived on the scene. She was shouting and screaming, no one could understand her, and assaulted the police when they were called. Currently in the cells, not speaking, looking very depressed. Dirty and thin, police surgeon suspects toxic confusional state, requests admission under Section 2 of the Mental Health Act, thinks police will then drop charges. Agreed: pt. to brought up to be seen, meanwhile contact Dr Weinstein for current care plans and duty social worker.

RKD (Reg.)

8.10.89 10.30 am. Before I had heard about the above episode from Dr Dorset, I met patient's daughter, Mrs Katewicz, coming to the hospital with a male friend. She was very distressed, I did not immediately recognise her which caused some antagonism. Apparently she arrived home last night late when neighbours told her her mother had been arrested.

Said, 'It's all my fault – I hate myself, I hate everybody'. The friend introduced himself as Mr Jakes, a senior master at Maria's school and said he had been with Maria last night. Maria: 'You might as well tell him, it'll all come out, we have been having an affair for months'. Mr Jakes is separated from his wife, awaiting a divorce and wants to marry Maria. He seems a very affectionate and supportive man: 'I'm sorry Mary is so upset, doctor, but in a way I'm glad things have come to a head, because now they'll have to take Mary's mother away where she can be properly looked after, Mary's had a Hell of a life, last night was the first time she has been out for months'.

When I said that it might or might not be possible to admit her compulsorily and in any case such detention would not be permanent, Maria broke down again and cried angrily, 'I won't take her back . . . I can't stand her anymore . . . you don't want to help us because you think we're just immigrants, I was born here . . . I hate all bloody Poles . . . why won't you put her away . . . if you won't admit her, you'll have to admit me, I can't stand any more of it'.

KWW (Cons.)

12.00 Mrs Z on ward. Just started seeing her. Telephone call from a Mr Peter Wilson who introduced himself as Mrs Z's son from Leeds. Said he had written to KWW but had not had a reply. Had brought his wife and children over this morning to visit his mother, neighbours told him about last night. Wants to come up to hospital immediately 'to find out what's going on'.

(RKD)

Case study D: (10)

Social Report on Mrs Katarina Zbigniewski

d.o.b. 27.10.1919

I visited this client by appointment in her home on 21st September, 1989 in the morning.

At first Mrs Zbigniewski was reluctant to let me in (I believe that a Polish speaking officer from the local authority posed rather a threat on her). However, when I explained the purpose of my visit, she relaxed and even offered me a cup of coffee and a cake in the middle of the interview.

History

Mrs Zbigniewski was the youngest in a family of seven children. Father was peasant and leased a three-hectare farm from the local country squire. Mother died when Katarina was four years of age, and consequently she was brought up by her older sister, who became 'like a Mother' to them all. Like all the children in the village she had the basic education of four classes of a country school. Father could not afford to send her to higher education in town. Up to the outbreak of war she lived in her village which firstly came under Russian occupation and then German. By a miracle father and older brother Kazimier were not deported to Russia. But Katarina was forcibly taken away by the Germans to Germany in 1940. There she worked on a farm, but later was placed in a munitions factory, where hard labour and inadequate living conditions in the camp made her so ill that she was nearly sent to be 'finished off' in a concentration camp. (Mrs Zbigniewski had TB before the war, which was treated inadequately). She had been examined by a factory doctor who had the power of 'life and death' over the inmates of the camp. Somehow she managed to persuade the foreman in the factory that her TB was not in an advanced stage, who in turn pleaded with the doctor.

After the war when the Polish territory where her village was situated was annexed to the Soviet Union she took the opportunity to come to Britain as a volunteer worker. In Britain, namely Bradford, she got a job in a mill. She was pleased to be among Polish people, and as soon as her husband proposed she decided to marry him. At work she did have problems with the supervisor, who was biased towards local girls and took advantage of Mrs Zbigniewski's lack of English.

Unfortunately, life at home was not better. She had been surprised when her husband proposed as he had been a famous soldier. He used to be helpful and caring at first, but in the last ten years he had become rather difficult. He had a drinking problem ('but Poles do like a drink, don't they?'); that was not too bad. She became upset when he abused her verbally and physically ('maybe it was due to his illness?'). The situation became unbearable when the children grew up and refused to be ruled by a rather narrow-minded father, who enforced on them a 'Polish' way of life.

Present

They had worked very hard to buy their present home. It was with pride that she told me how she and her husband saved the first £500 for a deposit; this home was their pride and joy. When the area deteriorated people who were better off financially moved away, it is only the old who stay behind. The black community took everything over. Children play on the back street, 'bombing' the garage with stones; the mosque across the road had bars at the windows, which reminds her very much of the barracks in the labour camps she was in in Germany. She feels unsafe going out alone.

Children

As far as her children are concerned Mrs Zbigniewski cares very much for her daughter, who is her pride and joy. She has invested everything in her – Maria is a teacher, hard working and helpful at home. ?She likes to go out occasionally (maybe too often ?) She said rather doubtfully that she hoped Maria would marry again but that she did not seem interested. Mrs Zbigniewski worries that Maria is in danger in the neighbourhood after dark; 'you know what they can do to white women'. Peter on the other hand married too soon, his wife is not what Mrs Zbigniewski wanted her daughter-in-law to be. She has lost him now, even his name is not the same (apparently Peter changed his name to that of his wife's family).

If only Peter had listened to her when he was at home. Mrs Zbigniewski feels rejected by her son, who insists on speaking English to her and will not reply when addressed in Polish. How can her son forget the fourth commandment? If only she had her mother; her mother died when she was four (Mrs Zbigniewski became rather tearful at this juncture).

Outside interests

Mrs Zbigniewski has few outlets outside the home. She attends church with two other Polish ladies. The Polish shop down the road still operates, but Maria prefers to do her shopping in Morrisons. She had only been outside Bradford once in the last five years to make a pilgrimage to Lourdes in France; even then she had problems with her travel document which was not in order and she was kept waiting by the immigration authorities for two hours at the port of entry.

Summary

Mrs Zbigniewski has had a difficult childhood, even more difficult years during the war, and the last ten years of her marriage have been rather stormy. Her problems with neighbours, people in authority, and her own children, seem to be genuine. When she is left in peace she remains 'locked in' her own world, but the least interference from outside and Mrs Zbigniewski hits back, totally misjudging the situation. This will be due to paranoia, perhaps more, I believe, to circumstances of a person who has been uprooted and thrown in the depths and found no stable base.

Even her nearest and dearest are against her. She cannot change her background, Polish ancestry or beliefs. She is trapped.

Dynamic formulation: narcissistic regression to paranoid–schizoid position; she identifies herself with her bad mother 'with a lot' of ego boundaries.

Gentle persuasion for her to attend community 'Polish Group' could break the isolation, and allow Mrs Zbigniewski to share her problems with others. Not suitable for psychotherapy.

Case study D: (11)

Memo

3.10.89.   3.30 pm

Message from switchboard: there is a soldier at reception who says his name is Kateswich, demanding to see someone about his grandmother.

References and Further Reading

Note:
An introductory set of works in transcultural psychiatry and intercultural therapy is suggested in the asterisked items, some of which are not otherwise cited in this volume.

Abel, T.M. and Metraux, R. (1974) *Culture and Psychotherapy*. New Haven: College and University Press.

*Ablon, J. (1980) The Significance of Cultural Patterning for the Alcoholic Family. *Family Process* **19**, 127-44.

*Abramowitz, S.I. and Murray, J. (1983) Race Effects in Psychotherapy. In Murray, J. and Abramson P. R. (Eds), *Bias in Psychotherapy*, New York: Praeger. pp 215-55.

Acharyya, S. and Moorhouse, S. (1987) Retrospective Study of One Hundred Cases: Profile of Patients Referred to Nafsiyat. (Unpublished ms.)

Acharyya, S., Moorhouse, S., Kareem, J. and Littlewood, R. (1989) Nafsiyat: A Psychotherapy Centre for Ethnic Minorities. *Psychiatric Bulletin* **13**, 358-60.

Acharyya, S., Moorhouse, S., Kareem, J. and Littlewood, R. (1989) An Evaluation of the Nafsiyat Centre for Ethnic and Cultural Minorities. (Unpublished ms.)

*Adebimpe, V.R. (1984) American Blacks and Psychiatry. *Transcultural Psychiatric Research Review*, **21**, 83-111.

Agger, I. and Jensen, S.B. (1989) Couples in Exile. Political Consciousness as an Element in the Psychosexual Dynamics of a Latin American Refugee Couple. *Sexual and Marital Therapy* **4** (1); 1-8.

*Allport J. (1986) *Psychoanalysis and Women*. New York: The Analytic Press.

Alibhai-Brown, Y. and Montague, A. (1992) *The Colour of Love*. London, Virago.

American Psychiatric Association (1980) Diagnostic and Statistical Manual of Mental Disorders. 3rd edn. Washington: American Psychiatric Association.

American Psychiatric Association (1987) Diagnostic and Statistical Manual of Mental Disorders. 3rd edn. Revised. Washington: American Psychiatric Association.

Amnesty International (1975) *Report on Torture*. New York: Farrar, Straus and Giroux.

Amnesty International (1984) *Torture in the Eighties*. London: Amnesty International Publications.

André, J. (1987) *L'Inceste Focale dans La Famille Noire Antillaise*. Paris: PUF.

Andreassen, D. (1989) Refugees and Asylum Seekers Coming to Europe Today. In *Refugees – The Trauma of Exile: The Humanitarian Role of Red Cross and Red Crescent*. Dordrecht; Martinus Nighoff.

Anwar, M. and Ali, A. (1987) *Overseas Doctors: Experience and Expectations*. London: Commission for Racial Equality.

Backett, K.C. (1982) *Mothers and Fathers: A Study of the Development and Negotiation of Parental Behaviour*. New York: Macmillan.

Bal, S. (1984) The Symptomatology of Mental Illness Among Asians in the West Midlands. BA Dissertation, Department of Economics and Social Sciences, Woverhampton Polytechnic.

Ballard, R. (1983) The Implications of Cultural Diversity for Medical Practice. (Unpublished ms.)

Ballhatchet, K. (1980) *Race, Sex and Class Under the Raj*. London: Weidenfeld and Nicolson.

Barker, J. (1984) *Black and Asian Old People in Britain*. Mitcham: Age Concern.

Baron, C. (1987) *Asylum to Anarchy*. London: Free Association Books.

*Barot, R. (1988) Social Anthropology, Ethnicity and Family Therapy. *Journal of Family Therapy*, **10**, 271–82.

Bateson, G. (1958) *Naven*. Stanford: Stanford University Press.

Bateson, G. (1973) *Steps to an Ecology of Mind*. St Albans: Paladin.

Bavington, J. (1984) A Frontier Mental Health Venture. Paper presented to 5th International Conference of Pakistan Psychiatric Society, Peshawar. (Copies available from Dr J. Bavington, Lynfield Mount Hospital, Bradford).

Bavington, J. (1987) The Stress which Leads to Distress. Paper presented to 4th Pakistan Psychiatric Society's International Conference, Islamabad. (Copies available from Dr J. Bavington, Lynfield Mount Hospital, Bradford.)

Bavington, J. and Majid, A. (1986) Psychiatric Services for Ethnic Minority Groups. In Cox *op cit*.

Beail, N. (1983) The Psychology of Fatherhood. *Bulletin of the British Psychological Society* **36**, 312–14.

Beck, J. (1987) *The Counsellor and the Black/White Relationship*. Boston: Houghton Mifflin.

*Beliappa, J. (1991) *Illness or Distress? Alternative Models of Mental Health*. London: Confederation of Indian Organisations.

Bernal, M. (1987) *Black Athena*, **1**. London: Free Association Press.

Bernstein, B. (1974) *Class, Codes and Control*. London: Routledge and Kegan Paul.

*Bettelheim, B. (1983) *Freud and Man's Soul*. London: Hogarth Press.

Bhat, A. *et al.* (1984) Psychiatric Workers as Emotional Beings: The Emotional Reactions of Staff following the Brixton Riots. *International Journal of Social Psychiatry*, **30**, 9–14.

Bick, E. (1967) The Experience of the Skin in Early Object Relations. *International Journal of Psychoanalysis*, **49**, 484.

Bion, W.R. (1984) *Learning from Experience*. London: Maresfield.

Bion, W.R. (1984) *Attention and Interpretation*. London: Maresfield.

Bloch, S. (1982) Psychotherapy. In Granville-Grossman, K. (Ed) *Recent Advances in*

Psychotherapy, 4. Edinburgh: Churchill Livingstone.

*Block, C. (1981) Black Americans and the Cross-Cultural Counselling and Psychotherapy Experience. In Marsella and Pedersen *op cit.*

Bochner, S. (Ed) (1982) *The Social Psychology of Cross-Cultural Relations – Cultures in Contact.* Oxford: Pergamon Press.

Bott, E. (1957) *Family and Social Networks.* London: Tavistock.

Bott, E. (1972) Psychoanalysis and Ceremony. In La Fontaine, J.S. (Ed) *The Interpretation of Ritual.* London: Tavistock.

*Bouras, N. and Littlewood, R. (Eds) (1988) Stress and Coping in the Greek Communities in Britain. Guy's Hospital (ms).

Bouras, N. Brough, D.I., Watson, P.J. (1982) Mental Health Advice Centre: Three Years of Experience. Research Report No. 1. Guy's Hospital (ms).

Bouras, N., Tufnell, G., Brough, D.I. and Watson, P.J. (1983) Mental Health Advice Centre. The Crisis Intervention Team Research Report No. 2. Guy's Hospital (ms).

Bourdieu, P. (1972) *Esquisse d'une Théorie de la Practique.* Genève: Librarie Droz.

Bowman, H.A. (1965) The Nature of Mental Health. In Sutherland, B. and Smith, B.K. (Eds) *Understanding Mental Health.* New York: Van Nostrand Reinhold.

Bremner, C. (1991) Saddam's Psyche and Paranoia under Intense Stress. London: *The Times,* January 17.

*Brent Irish Mental Health Group (1986) *The Irish Experience of Mental Ill Health in London.* London: Brent Irish Mental Health Group.

*British Association of Social Workers (1982) *Social Work in Multi-Cultural Britain.* London: British Association of Social Workers.

Brown, D. and Pedder, J. (1980) *Introduction to Psychotherapy.* London: Tavistock.

Burke, A. (Ed) (1984) Racism and Mental Illness, *International Journal of Social Psychiatry,* Special Issue, **30**, (1 and 2).

Callaway, H. (1987) *Gender, Culture and Empire: European Women in Colonial Nigeria.* London: Macmillan.

Calley, M.J.C. (1965) *God's People: West Indian Pentecostal Sects in England.* Oxford: Oxford University Press.

Campling, P. (1989) Race, Culture and Psychotherapy. *Psychiatric Bulletin* **13**, 550–51.

Caplan, G. (1970) *The Theory and Practice of Mental Health Consultation.* London: Tavistock.

*Carkhuff, R.R. and Pierce, R. (1967) Differential Effects of Therapist Race and Social Class upon Patient Depth of Self Exploration in the Initial Interview. *Journal of Consulting and Clinical Psychology,* **31**, 632–44.

Carothers, J.C. (1972) *The Mind of Man in Africa.* London: Stacey.

Carstairs, M. (1973) Psychiatric Training for Foreign Medical Graduates. In Forrest, A. *Companion to Psychiatric Studies.* Edinburgh: Churchill-Livingstone.

Carstairs, M. and Kapur, R.L. (1976) *The Great Universe of Koto: Stress, Change and Mental Disorder in an Indian Village.* London: Hogarth.

Carter, H.J.H. (1979) Frequent Mistakes Made with Black Patients in Psychotherapy. *Journal of the National Medical Association,* **71**, 1007–13.

Casse, P. (1981) *Training for the Cross-Cultural Mind. A Handbook for Cross-Cultural Trainers and Consultants.* Washington: Society for Intercultural Education.

Chakraborty, A. (1990) *Social Stress and Mental Health: A Social Psychiatric Field Study of*

Calcutta. New Delhi: Sage.

Chandrasena, R. (1983) The Use of Traditional Therapies by Ethnic Minorities in the U.K. Typescript. (Abstracted in *Transcultural Psychiatric Research Review*, **20**, 297–9).

Chiappe, M., Lemlij, M. and Millones, L. (1985) *Alucinogenos y Shamanismo en el Peru Contemporaneo.* Lima: Virrey.

Cienfuegos, A.J. and Monelli, C. (1983) The Testimony of Political Repression as a Therapeutic Instrument. *American Journal of Orthopsychiatry*, **53**, 43–51.

Clark, J. and Lago, C. (1980) Personal Values in Relation to Ethnic Minority Clients. *Counselling News*, **32**, 21–4.

*Cochrane, R. (1983). *The Social Creation of Mental Illness.* New York: Longman.

Cochrane, R., and Stopes-Roe, M. (1977) Psychological and Social Adjustment of Asian Immigrants to Britain: A Community Survey. *Social Psychiatry*, **12**, 195–207.

Cocks, G. (1985) *Psychotherapy in the Third Reich.* New York: Oxford University Press.

Cohen, N. (1982) Same or Different? A Pattern of Identity in Cross-Cultural Marriages. *Journal of Family Therapy*, **4**, 177–99.

Collomb, H. (1973) L'Avenir de la Psychiatrie en Afrique. *Psychopathologie Africaine*, **9**, 343–70.

*Coltart, N. (1986) Slouching Towards Bethlehem: Thinking the Unthinkable in Psychoanalysis. In Kohon, G. (Ed) *The British School of Psychoanalysis: The Independent Tradition.* London: Free Association Books.

*Comas-Diaz, L. and Griffith, E.E.H. (Eds) (1987) *Clinical Guidelines in Cross-Cultural Mental Health.* New York: Wiley.

*Combs, D. (1978) *Crossing Culture in Therapy.* New York: Brooks.

Commission for Racial Equality (1985) *A Report on the Seminar on Racism Awareness Training.* London: Commission for Racial Equality.

Commission for Racial Equality (1988) *Report of a Formal Investigation into St George's Hospital Medical School.* London: Commission for Racial Equality.

Commission for Racial Equality (1990) *Annual Report.* London: Commission for Racial Equality.

Cooklin, A. (1982) Position Statement in Family Therapy. (Unpublished ms.)

Cooper, D. (1971) *The Death of the Family.* London: Allen Lane.

Corin, E. and Bibeau, G. (1980) Psychiatric Perspectives in Africa: 2, *Transcultural Psychiatric Research Review*, **16**, 147–78.

*Cox, S. (Ed) (1986) *Transcultural Psychiatry.* London: Croom Helm.

Crapanzano, V. (1973) *The Hamadsha: A Study in Moroccan Ethnopsychiatry.* Berkeley: University of California Press.

*Curry, A. (1964) Myth, Transference and the Black Psychotherapist. *International Review of Psychoanalysis*, **45**.

Danforth, L.M. (1989) *Firewalking and Religious Healing: The Anastenaria of Greece and the American Firewalking Movement.* Princeton: Princeton University Press.

*D'Ardenne, P. and Mahtani, A. (1989) *Transcultural Counselling in Action.* London: Sage.

Dayal, M. (1987) Psychotherapy Services For Black People in the NHS – A Psychotherapist's View (Unpublished ms.)

Deleuze, G. and Guattari, F. (1984) *Anti-Oedipus: Capitalism and Schizophrenia.* London: Athlone Press.

Devereux, G. (1970) *Essais d'Ethnopsychiatrie Genérale*. Paris: Gallimard.

*Devereux, G. (1978) Ethnopsychoanalysis. Berkeley: California.

De Zulueta, F. (1984) The Implications of Bilingualism in the Study of Treatment of Psychiatric Disorder. *Psychological Medicine*, **14**, 541–57.

*Dinicola, V.F. (1985) Family Therapy and Transcultural Psychiatry: An Emerging Synthesis. *Transcultural Psychiatric Research Review*, **22**, 81–113 and 151–81.

Dinicola, V.F. (1986) Beyond Babel: Family Therapy as a Cultural Translation. *International Journal of Family Therapy*, **7**, 179–91.

Dolan, B. *et al* (1991) Addressing Racism in Therapy: Is The Therapeutic Community Model Applicable? *International Journal of Social Psychiatry*, 37, 71–9.

Donovan, J. (1986) *We Don't Buy Sickness: It Just Comes: Health, Illness and Health Care in the Lives of Black People in London*. London: Gower.

Dow, J. (1986) Universal Aspects of Symbolic Healing: A Theoretical Synthesis. *American Anthropologist*, **88**, 56–69.

*Draguns, J.G. (1975) Resocialisation into Culture: The Complexities of Taking A Worldwide View of Psychotherapy. In Brislin, R.W., Bochner, S. and Conner, W.J. (Eds) *Cross-Cultural Perspectives on Learning*. New York: Sage.

Dumont, L. (1966) *Homo Hierarchicus*. Paris: Gallimard.

Edgell, S. (1980) *Middle Class Couples*. London: Allen and Unwin.

Eichenbaum, L. and Orbach, S. (1982) *Outside in: Inside out*. Harmondsworth: Penguin.

Eisenbruch, M. (1984) Cross-Cultural Aspects of Bereavement I: A Conceptual Framework for Comparative Analysis. *Culture, Medicine and Psychiatry*, **8**, 283–309.

Eisenbruch, M. (1984) Cross Cultural Aspects of Bereavement II: Ethnic and Cultural Variations in the Development of Bereavement Practices. *Culture, Medicine and Psychiatry*, **8**, 315–47.

Eisenbruch, M. (1989) Medical Education for a Multicultural Society. *Medical Journal of Australia*, **151**, 574–80.

Ekman, P. and Friesen, W. (1971) Constants Across Cultures in Face and Emotion. *Journal of Personality and Social Psychology*, **17**, 124–29.

Eliade, M. (1964) *Shamanism*. Princeton: Princeton University Press.

El Islam, M.F. (1969) Depression and Guilt: A Study at an Arab Psychiatric Clinic. *Social Psychiatry*, **2** 56–8.

Ellen, R. (1988) Fetishism. *Man*, **23**, 213–35.

Ellison, R. (1956) *Invisible Man*. Harmondsworth: Penguin.

Epstein, A.L. (1978) *Ethos and Identity*. London: Tavistock.

Erikson, E. (1959) *Identity in the Life Cycle*. New York: Norton.

*Erikson, E. (1965) *Childhood and Society*. Harmondsworth: Penguin.

Ernst, S. and Maguire, M. (1987) *Living with the Sphinx*. London: The Women's Press.

*Eysenck, H.J. (1952) The Effects of Psychotherapy: An Evaluation. *Journal of Consulting Psychology*, **16**, 319–24.

*Falicov, C. (1983) *Cultural Perspectives in Family Therapy*. Rockville: Aspen.

Falicov, C. and Carter E.A. (1980) Cultural Variations in the Family Life Cycle. In Carter, E.A. and McGoldrick, M. (Eds) *The Family Life Cycle: A Framework for Family Therapy*. New York: Gardner Press.

*Feifil, H. and Eels, J. (1963) Patients and Therapists Assess the Same Psychotherapy. *Journal of Consulting Psychology*, **27** (4), 310–18.

Fernando, S (1991) *Mental Health, Race and Culture*. London: Macmillan.

Firth, R. (1961) Suicide and Risk Taking in Tikopia Society. *Psychiatry*, **2**, 1–17.

Firth, R. (1969) *Essays on Social Organization and Values*, London: The Athlone Press.

Firth, R. (Ed) (1956) *Two Studies of Kinship in London*. London School of Economics Monographs on Social Anthropology, **15**, London: The Athlone Press.

*Fisher, L.G. (1985) *Colonial Madness: Mental Health in the Barbadian Social Order*. New Jersey: Rutgers University Press.

Foley, V.D. (1982) Family Therapy with Black, Disadvantaged Families. In Gurman, A.S. (Ed) *Questions and Answers in the Practice of Family Therapy*. New York: Brunner/ Mazel.

Fortes, M. (1983) *Oedipus and Job in West African Religion*, 2nd edn. Cambridge: Cambridge University Press.

*Frank, J. (1961) *Persuasion and Healing: A Comparative Study of Psychotherapy*. New York: Schoken.

Freud, S.: Standard Edition (Translated by James Strachey). London: The Hogarth Press. Institute of Psychoanalysis.

*Fromm, E. (1956) *The Sane Society*. London: Routledge and Kegan Paul.

Fromm, E. (1957) *The Art of Loving*. London: Allen and Unwin.

*Fromm, E. (1960) *The Fear of Freedom*. London: Routledge and Kegan Paul.

Fromm, E. (1973) *The Crisis of Psychoanalysis*. Harmondsworth: Penguin.

Fromm, E. (1986) *Psychoanalysis and Buddhism*. London: Unwin.

Frosh, S. (1987) *The Politics of Psychoanalysis*. London: Macmillan Education.

Frosh, S. (1989) Psychoanalysis and Racism. In Richards, B., *Crisis of the Self: Further Essays on Psychoanalysis and Politics*. London: Free Association Books.

*Furnham, A. and Bochner, S. (1986) *Culture Shock, Psychological Reactions to Unfamiliar Environments*. London: Methuen.

Gallessich, J. (1982) *The Profession and Practice of Consultation*. London: Jossey Bass.

Gardiner, M. (1972) *The Wolf Man and Sigmund Freud*, London: Hogarth.

*Garfield, S.L. and Bergin, A.E. (1986) *Handbook of Psychotherapy and Behaviour Change*, 3rd edn. New York: Wiley.

Gaw, A. (Ed) (1982) *Cross-Cultural Psychiatry*. Boston: Wright.

Gay, P. (1987) *A Godless Jew: Freud, Atheism and the Making of Psychoanalysis*. New Haven: Yale University Press.

Geertz, C. (1973) *The Interpretation of Cultures*. New York: Basic Books.

Gelder, M., Gath, D., and Mayou, R. (1985) *Oxford Textbook of Psychiatry*. Oxford: Oxford University Press.

Geller, J.D. (1988) Racial Bias in the Evaluation of Patients for Psychotherapy. In Comas-Diaz and Griffith *op cit*.

Gellner, E. (1985) *The Psychoanalytic Movement*. London: Paladin.

Gilman, S. (1985) *Difference and Psychopathology: Stereotypes of Sexuality, Race and Madness*. Ithaca: Cornell University Press.

Gluckman, M. (1963) *Order and Rebellion in Tribal Africa*. London: Cohen and West.

Goldberg, D. (1978) *Manual of the General Health Questionnaire*. Windsor: National

Federation for Educational Research – Nelson.

Goldfeld, A.E., Mollica, R.F., Pesavento, B.H. and Faraone, S.U. (1988) The Physical and Psychological Sequelae of Torture – Symptomatology and Diagnosis. *Journal of the American Medical Association,* **259** (18), 2725–9.

Goodchild, M.E. and Duncan-Jones, P. (1985) Chronicity and the General Health Questionnaire. *British Journal of Psychiatry,* **146,** 55–61.

Gorrell Barnes, G. (1982) Pattern and Intervention: Research Findings and the Development of Family Therapy Theory. In Bentovim, A. *et al.* (Eds) *Family Therapy: Complementary Frameworks of Theory and Practice,* **1.** London: Academic Press.

Graccus, F. (1980) Les Lieux de la Mère dans Les Sociétés Afro-Americaines. Paris: CARÉ.

Greben, S.E. (1981) The Essence of Psychotherapy. *British Journal of Psychiatry,* **138,** 449–55.

*Grier, W.H. and Cobbs, P.M. (1969) *Black Rage.* London: Cape.

Griffith, E.E.H. and Young, S.L. (1988) A Cross-Cultural Introduction to the Therapeutic Aspects of Christian Religious Ritual. In Comas-Diaz and Griffith *op cit.*

Griffith, M.S. and Jones, E.E. (1979) Race and Psychotherapy: Changing Perspectives. *Current Psychiatric Therapies,* **16,** 225–35.

*Grinberg, L. and Grinberg, R. (1989) *Psychoanalytic Perspectives on Migration and Exile.* New Haven: Yale University Press.

Grove, D. and Panzer, B. (1989) *Resolving Traumatic Memories: Metaphors and Symbols in Psychotherapy.* New York: Norton.

Gurman, A.S. (1982) Creating a Therapeutic Alliance in Marital Therapy. In Gurman, A.S. (Ed) *Questions and Answers in the Practice of Family Therapy.* New York: Brunner/Mazel.

Gurman, A.S. and Kniskern, D.P. (1981) Family Therapy Outcome Research: Knowns and Unknowns. In Gurman, A.S. and Kniskern, D.P. (Eds) *Handbook of Family Therapy.* New York: Brunner/Mazel.

Guthrie, R.V. (1975) *Even the Rat was White: A Historical View of Psychology.* New York: Harper and Row.

Halifax, J. (1980) *Shamanic Voices.* Harmondsworth: Penguin.

Haraway, D. (1989) *Primate Visions: Gender, Race and Nature in the World of Modern Science.* New York: Routledge.

*Harding, T.W. (1976) Validating a Method of Psychiatric Case Identification in Jamaica. *Bulletin of the World Health Organisation,* **54,** (2), 225–31.

Harré, R. (1983) *Personal Being: A Theory of Individual Psychology.* Oxford: Basil Blackwell.

Harris, C. (1957) Possession 'Hysteria' in a Kenya Tribe. *American Anthropologist,* **59,** 1046–66.

*Harrison, D. (1975) Race as a Counsellor-Client Variable in Counselling and Psychotherapy: A Review of Research. *The Counselling Psychologist,* **5** (1), 124–33.

Harrison, G., Owens, D., Holton, A., Neilon, D. and Boot, D. (1988): A Prospective Study of Severe Mental Disorder in Afro-Caribbean Patients. *Psychological Medicine,* **18;** 643–58.

*Heelas, P. and Lock, A. (Eds) (1981) *Indigenous Psychologies: The Anthropology of the Self*. London: Academic Press.

*Helman, C. (1985) *Culture, Health and Illness*. Bristol: Wright.

*Henriques, F. (1974) *Children of Caliban*. London: Secker and Warburg.

*Hernton, C.C. (1969) *Sex and Racism*. London: Deutsch.

Herz, F. (1982) Ethnic Differences and Family Therapy. In Gurman, A.S. (Ed) *Questions and Answers in the Practice of Family Therapy*, **2**., New York: Brunner/Mazel.

Hickling, F.W. (1988) Politics and the Psychotherapy Context. In Comas-Diaz and Griffith *op cit*.

Hipgrave, T. (1982) Lone Fatherhood: A Problematic Status. In McKee, L. and O'Brien, M. (Eds) *The Father Figure*. London: Tavistock.

*Ho, M.K. (1987) *Family Therapy with Ethnic Minorities*. California: Sage.

Hobson, R.E. (1986) *Forms of Feeling: The Heart of Psychotherapy*. London: Tavistock.

Hodes, M. (1985) Family Therapy and the Problem of Cultural Relativism: A Reply to Dr Lau. *Journal of Family Therapy*, **7**, 261–72.

*Hodes, M. (1989) Annotation: Culture and Family Therapy. *Journal of Family Therapy*, **11**, 117–28.

Hoggart, R. (1957) *The Uses of Literacy*. Harmondsworth: Penguin.

Hook, R.H. (Ed) (1979) *Fantasy and Symbol: Studies in Anthropological Interpretation*. London: Academic Press.

Horowitz, M.J. (1976). *Stress Response Syndromes*. New York: Jason Aronson.

Horton, R. (1983) Social Psychologies: African and Western. In Fortes, M. *op cit*.

Howell, S. (1981) Rules Not Words. In Heelas, P. and Lock, A. (Eds) *op cit*.

Huby, G. and Salkind, M.R. (1990) *Journal of Social Work Practice*, **4** (2) 90–7.

Hughes, C.C. (1985) Culture-bound or Construct-bound? The Syndromes and DSM-III. In Simons R.C. and Hughes C.C. *op cit*.

Hutton, F. (1985) Self Referrals to a Community Mental Health Centre: A Three Year Study. *British Journal of Psychiatry*, **147**, 540–44.

Hyam, R. (1990) *Empire and Sexuality: The British Experience*. Manchester: Manchester University Press.

Ikechukwu, S.T.C. (1989) Approaches to Psychotherapy in Africans: Do They Have to be Non-Medical? *Culture, Medicine and Psychiatry*, **13**, 419–35.

Ilahi, N. (1989) Psychotherapy Services to the Ethnic Communities. Ealing Health Authority.

Ineichen, B., Harrison, G. and Morgan, M.S. (1984) Psychiatric Hospital Admissions in Bristol. *British Journal of Psychiatry*, **145**, 600–11.

Jaffa, T. (1992) Therapy with Families Who have Experienced Torture. In Wilson, J. and Raphael, B. (Eds) *Handbook of Traumatic Stress*. New York: Plenum.

Jalali, B. (1988) Ethnicity, Cultural Adjustment and Behaviour: Implications for Family Therapy. In Comas-Diaz and Griffith, *op cit*.

Janet, P. (1925) *Psychological Healing: A Historical and Clinical Study*. London: Allen and Unwin.

Jansen, J.M. (1978) *The Quest for Therapy: Medical Pluralism in Lower Zaire*. Berkeley: University of California Press.

Jensen, S.B. and Agger, I. (1988) The Testimony Method: The use of Testimony as a Psychotherapeutic Tool in the Treatment of Traumatized Refugees in Denmark. Paper presented at the First European Conference on Traumatic Stress Studies, Lincoln, England.

Johnstone, A. and Goldberg, D. (1976) Psychiatric Screening in General Practice. *Lancet*, **1**, 605–8.

Jones, A. and Seagull, A.A. (1977) Dimensions of the Relationship between the Black Patient and the White Therapist. A Theoretical Overview. *American Psychologist*, **32**, 850–69.

Jones, E.E. (1978) Effects of Race on Psychotherapy Process and Outcome: An Exploratory Investigation. *Psychotherapy*, **15**, 226–36.

*Kakar, S. (1978) *The Inner World: A Psychoanalytic Study of Childhood and Society in India.* New York and Delhi: Oxford University Press.

*Kakar, S. (1982) *Shamans, Mystics and Doctors: A Psychological Inquiry into India and its Healing Traditions.* Delhi: Oxford University Press.

*Kakar, S. (1985) Psychoanalysis and Non Western Culture. *International Review of Psychoanalysis*, **12**, 441–5.

Kanishige, E. (1973). Cultural Factors in Group Counselling and Interaction. *Personnel and Guidance Journal*, **51** (6), 407.

Kapo, R. (1981) *A Savage Culture.* London: Quartet.

Karasu, T.B. (1985). Quoted in Bergin, S. and Garfield, A.E. (1986). *Handbook of Psychotherapy and Behaviour Change* 3rd edn. New York: Wiley, p. 24.

Kareem, J. (1978) Conflicting Concepts of Mental Health in Multi-Cultural Society. *Psychiatrica Clinica*, **11**, 90–95.

Kareem, J. (1987) Clinical Director's Address. In Proceedings of Conference on Assessment and Treatment Across Cultures. London: Nafsiyat, pp. 9–14.

Kareem, J. (1988) Outside In – Inside Out: Some Considerations in Inter-Cultural Therapy. *Journal of Social Work Practice*, **3** (3), 57–77.

Kaslow, F.D. (1982) Working with Families Cross-Culturally. In Gurman, A.S. (Ed), *Questions and Answers in the Practice of Family Therapy*, **2**, New York: Brunner/Mazel.

Katnelson, I. (1973) *Black Men, White Cities.* Oxford: Oxford University Press.

*Kernberg, O.F., Burskin, E., Coyne, L., Appelbaum, A., Horowitz, L and Voth, H. (1972) Psychotherapy and Psychoanalysis: Final Report of the Menninger Foundation's Psychotherapy Research Project. *Bulletin of the Menninger Clinic.* **36**, Nos. 1 and 2.

*Kiev, A. (Ed) (1964a) *Magic, Faith and Healing.* New York: Free Press.

Kiev, A. (Ed) (1964b) Psychotherapeutic Aspects of Pentecostal Sects among West Indian Immigrants to England. *British Journal of Sociology*, **15**, 129–38.

Kiev, A. (1968) *Curandismo: Mexican Folk Psychiatry.* New York: Free Press.

King, Patricia, (1982) Racial and Cultural Factors in A Casework Relationship. In Cheetham, J. (Ed) *Social Work and Ethnicity.* London: Allen and Unwin.

King, Pearl, (1989) Activities of British Psychoanalysts During the Second World War and the Influence of their Inter-disciplinary Collaboration on the Development of Psychoanalysis in Great Britain. *International Review of Psychoanalysis*, **16**, 15–33.

Kinzie, J.D. (1985) Cultural Aspects of Psychiatric Treatment with Indo-Chinese

Refugees. *American Journal of Social Psychiatry*, **5**, 47–53.

Kitamura, T., Sugawara, M., Aoki, M. and Shima, S. (1989) Validity of the Japanese Version of the GHQ among Antenatal Clinic Attenders. *Psychological Medicine*, **19** (2), 507–11.

Klauber, J. (1986) *Difficulties in the Analytical Encounter*. London: Free Association Books (Maresfield Library).

Klein, E.B., Thomas, C.S. and Bellis, E.C. (1971) When Warring Groups Meet: The Use of a Group Approach in Police-Black Community Relations. *Social Psychiatry*, **6**, 93–9.

Klein, J. (1987) *Our Need For Others and its Roots in Infancy*. London: Tavistock.

Kleinman, A. (1987) Anthropology and Psychiatry: The Role of Culture in Cross-Cultural Research on Illness, *British Journal of Psychiatry*, **151**, 447–54.

*Kleinman, A. (1988) *Rethinking Psychiatry: From Cultural Category to Personal Experience*. New York: Free Press.

*Kleinman, A. and Good, B. (Eds) (1985) *Culture and Depression*. Berkeley: University of California Press.

*Kleinman, A. and Lin, T. (Eds) (1981) *Normal and Deviant Behaviour in Chinese Culture*. Dordrecht; Reidel.

Kleinman, A. and Sung, L.H. (1979) Why Do Indigenous Practitioners Successfully Heal? *Social Science and Medicine*, **13**, 7–26.

Klineberg, D. (1982) Contact between Ethnic Groups. A Historical Perspective of Some Aspects of Theory and Research. In Bocher, S. (Ed) *Cultures in Conflict*. Oxford: Pergamon Press.

*Koeter, M.W.J., Brink, W. van den and Ormel, J. (1989) Chronic Psychiatric Complaints and the General Health Questionnaire. *British Journal of Psychiatry*, **155**, 186–90.

*Kovel, J. (1988) *White Racism: A Psychohistory*: London: Free Association Books.

*Krause, B. (1989) The Sinking Heart: A Punjabi Communication of Distress. *Social Science and Medicine*, **29**, 563–75.

La Fontaine, J.S. (Ed) (1978) *Sex and Age as Principles of Social Differentiation*. London: Academic Press.

*Lago, C. (1981). Cross Cultural Counselling: Some Developments, Thoughts and Hypotheses. *New Community*, May 1981.

Laguerre, M.S. (1987) *Afro-Caribbean Folk Medicine*. Massachusetts: Bergin and Garvey.

Laing, R.D. and Esterson, A. (1974) *Sanity, Madness and the Family*. London: Tavistock.

Lambeth Social Services (1987) 'Whose Child' – Report on the Inquiry into the Death of Tyra Henry. London: LSS.

Lang, P.E. (1969) The Mechanics of Desensitization and the Laboratory Study of Fear. In Franks, C.M. (Ed) *Behaviour Therapy, Appraisal and Status*. New York: McGraw Hill.

Laslett, P. (1972) *Household and Family in Past Time*. Cambridge: Cambridge University Press.

Lattanzi, M., Galvan, U., Rizzetto, A., Gavioli, I. *et al.* (1988). Estimating Psychiatric Morbidity in the Community. Standardisation of the Italian Versions of GHQ and CIS. *Social Psychiatry and Psychiatric Epidemiology*, **23** (4), 267–72.

*Lau, A. (1984) Transcultural Issues in Family Therapy. *Journal of Family Therapy*, **6**, 91–112.

Laurence, M. (1987) *Fed up and Hungry*. London: The Women's Press.

Leach, E. (1976) *Culture and Communication*. Cambridge: Cambridge University Press.

Leff, S. (1981) *Psychiatry around the Globe: A Transcultural View*. New York: Dekker.

Levi, P. (1987). *Moments of Reprieve*. Harmondsworth: Penguin Group.

Lévi-Strauss, C. (1968a) The Sorcerer and his Magic. In Lévi-Strauss, *Structural Anthropology*, Harmondsworth: Penguin.

Lévi-Strauss, C. (1968b) *The Effectiveness of Symbols*. In Lévi-Strauss *op cit*.

*Lévi-Strauss, C. (1985) *The View From Afar*, Harmondsworth: Penguin.

Lewis, C. and O'Brien, M. (Eds) (1987) *Reassessing Fatherhood*. London: Sage.

Lewis, G. Croft-Jeffreys, C. and David, A. (1990) Are British Psychiatrists Racist? *British Journal of Psychiatry*, **157**, 410–15.

Lewis, I.M. (1966) Spirit Possession and Deprivation Cults. *Man*, **1**, 307–29.

Limentani, A.: (1986) Affects and Psychoanalytical Situation. In Kohon G. (Ed) *The British School of Psychoanalysis: The Independent Tradition*. London: Free Association Press.

*Littlewood, R. (1980) Anthropology and Psychiatry: An Alternative Approach, *British Journal of Medical Psychology*, **53**, 213–25.

Littlewood, R. (1983) The Antinomian Hasid. *British Journal of Medical Psychology*, **56**, 67–78.

Littlewood, R. (1984a) The Imitation of Madness: The Influence of Psychopathology upon Culture. *Social Science and Medicine*, **19**, 705–15.

Littlewood, R. (1984b) The Individual Articulation of Shared Symbols. *Journal of Operational Psychiatry*, **15**, 17–24.

Littlewood, R. (1986a) Russian Dolls and Chinese Boxes: An Anthropological Approach to the Implicit Models of Psychiatry. In Cox (1986) *op cit*.

Littlewood, R. (1986b) Ethnic Minorities and the Mental Health Act. Patterns of Explanation. *Bulletin of the Royal College of Psychiatrists*, **10**, 306–8.

Littlewood, R. (1988) From Vice to Madness: The Semantics of Naturalistic and Personalistic Understanding in Trinidad Local Medicine. *Social Science and Medicine*, **27**, 129–48.

Littlewood, R. (1989a) Science, Shamanism and Hermeneutics. *Anthropology Today*, **5** (1), 5–11.

Littlewood, R. (1989b). Glossary. In *Report of the Royal College of Psychiatrists Special (Ethnic Issues) Committee*. London: Royal College of Psychiatrists.

*Littlewood, R. (1990) From Categories to Contexts: A Decade of the 'New Cross-Cultural Psychiatry', *British Journal of Psychiatry*, **156**, 308–27.

*Littlewood, R. (1991) Against Pathology: The New Psychiatry and It's Critics. *British Journal of Psychiatry*, **159**, 696–702.

Littlewood, R. (1992a) Symptoms, Struggles and Functions: What Does Overdose Represent? In McDonald, M. (Ed) *Women and Drugs*. London: Berg.

Littlewood, R. (1992b) Culture and DSMIV: Is the Classification Internationally Valid? *Psychiatric Bulletin* (In press).

Littlewood, R. and Cross, S. (1980) Ethnic Minorities and Psychiatric Services. *Sociology of Health and Illness*, **2**, 194–201 (but see Milner, G. and Hayes, G. (1988)

Correspondence. *British Medical Journal*, **297**; 359).

Littlewood, R., and Lipsedge, M. (1981) Acute Psychotic Reactions in Caribbean-born Patients. *Psychological Medicine*, **11**, 303–18.

Littlewood, R., and Lipsedge, M. (1987) The Butterfly and the Serpent. *Culture Medicine and Psychiatry*, **11**; 289–335.

Littlewood, R., and Lipsedge, M. (1988) Psychiatric Illness Among British Afro-Caribbeans (Editorial). *British Medical Journal*, **296**, 950–1.

*Littlewood, R., and Lipsedge, M. (1989) *Aliens and Alienists: Ethnic Minorities and Psychiatry*. 2nd revised edn. London: Unwin Hyman (originally published 1982).

Lomas, P. (1987) *The Limits of Interpretation*. Harmondsworth: Penguin Books.

Loudon, J. (1959) Psychogenic Disorder and Social Conflict among the Zulu. In Opler, M.K. (Ed) *Culture and Mental Health*. New York: Macmillan.

Luborsky, L., Singer, B., and Luborsky, L. (1975) Comparative Studies of Psychotherapies. Is It True That 'Everyone Has Won and All Must Have Prizes'? *Archives of General Psychiatry*, **32**, 995–1008.

Macfarlane, A. (1978) *The Origins of British Individualism*. Edinburgh: Blackwood.

Madanes, C. (1982) *Strategic Family Therapy*, San Francisco: Jossey Bass.

Majid, A. (1986) Psychiatric Services for Ethnic Minority Groups. In Cox *op cit.*

Malan, D.H. (1975). *A Study of Brief Psychotherapy*. London: Plenum.

Malzberg, B. (1940) *Social and Biological Aspects of Mental Disease*. New York: Hogarth Press.

*Mannoni, O. (1964) *Prospero and Caliban: The Psychology of Colonisation*. New York: Praeger.

*Maranhão, T. (1984) Family Therapy and Anthropology. *Culture, Medicine and Psychiatry*, **8**, 255–79.

Maranhão, T. (1986) *Therapeutic Discourse and Socratic Dialogue*. Madison: University of Wisconsin Press.

Marcos, L.R. (1973) The Effect of Interview Language on Evaluation of Psychotherapies in Spanish American Patients. *American Journal of Psychiatry*, **130**, 549–53.

Marcos, L.R. (1988) Understanding Ethnicity in Psychotherapy with Hispanic Patients. *American Journal of Psychoanalysis*, **48** (1), 35–42.

*Marsella, A.J. and Pedersen, P.B. (Eds) (1981) *Cross-Cultural Counselling and Psychotherapy*. New York: Pergamon Press.

*Marsella, A.J. and White, G. (Eds) (1982) *Cultural Conceptions of Mental Health and Therapy*. Dordrecht: Reidel.

*Marsella, A.J. De Vos, G. and Hsu, F.L.K. (Eds) (1985) *Culture and Self: Asian and Western Perspectives*. London: Tavistock.

Mason, P. (1962) *Prospero's Magic*. London: Oxford University Press.

Masson, J. (1988) *Against Therapy*. Glasgow: Collins.

McGill, D. and Pearce, J.K. (1982) British Families. In McGoldrick, M. *et al.* (Eds) *op cit.*

McGoldrick, M., Pearce, J. and Giardino, J. (Eds) (1982) *Ethnicity and Family Therapy*. New York: Guildford Press.

McGovern, D. and Cope, R.V. (1987) The Compulsory Detention of Males of Different Ethnic Groups. *British Journal of Psychiatry*, **150**, 505–12.

McGrath, W.J. (1986) *Freud's Discovery of Psychoanalysis: The Politics of Hysteria*. Ithaca: Cornell University Press.

McKee, L. (1982) Fathers' Participation in Infant Care: A Critique. In McKee, L. and O'Brien, M. (Eds) *The Father Figure*. London: Tavistock.

McKee, L., and O'Brien, M. (Eds) (1982) *The Father Figure*. London: Tavistock.

*Mercer, K. (1986) Racism and Transcultural Psychiatry. In Miller, P. and Rose, N. (Eds) *The Power of Psychiatry*. London: Polity.

Miller, K. *et al*. (1983) Psychotherapists and the Process of Profession-Building. OPUS.

*Miller-Pietroni, M. (Ed) (1988) Intercultural Social Work and Psychotherapy. (Special Issue) *Journal of Social Work Practice*, **13**, No. 13.

Minuchin, S. (1977) *Families and Family Therapy*, London: Tavistock.

Minuchin, S. *et al*. (1967) *Families of the Slums*, New York: Basic Books.

Minuchin, S. *et al*. (1978) *Psychosomatic Families*, Cambridge, Mass: Harvard University Press.

Mitchell, J. (1984) *Women – The Longest Revolution*. London: Virago.

Mollica, R.F. (1987) The Trauma Story: The Psychiatric Care of Refugee Survivors of Violence and Torture. In Ochberg, F.M. (Ed) *Post-Traumatic Therapy and the Victims of Violence*. New York: Brunner/Mazel.

Mollica, R.F., Wyshak, G. and Lavelle, J. (1987) The Psycho-Social Impact of War, Trauma and Torture on South Eastern Asian Refugees. *American Journal of Psychiatry*, **144**, 1567–72.

Moodley, P. (1987) The Fanon Project: A Day Centre in Brixton. *Bulletin of the Royal College of Psychiatrists*, **11**, 417–18.

Moorhouse, S., Acharyya, S., Littlewood, R., and Kareem, J. (1989). An Evaluation of the Nafsiyat Psychotherapy Centre for Ethnic and Cultural Minorities. Report of a Three-Year Study Funded by the Department of Health and Social Security. (Unpublished ms.)

Mrazel, D. (1985) Child Psychiatric Consultation and Liaison to Paediatrics. In Rutter, M and Hersov, L., (Eds) *Child and Adolescent Psychiatry, Modern Approaches*. Oxford: Blackwell Scientific Publications.

Mullings, L. (1984) *Therapy, Ideology and Social Change: Mental Healing in Urban Ghana*. Berkeley: California University Press.

Munoz, L. (1980) Exile as Bereavement: Socio-Psychological Manifestations of Chilean Exiles in Great Britain. *British Journal of Medical Psychology*, **53**, 227–32.

Murphy, H.B.M. (1986) The Mental Health Impact of British Cultural Traditions. In Cox *op cit*.

Newsome, A., Thorne, J., and Wyld, K. (1975) *Student Counselling in Practice*, London: University of London Press.

Newson, E., and Newson, J. (1970) *Four Years Old in an Urban Community*. Harmondsworth: Penguin.

Newson, J., and Newson, E. (1963) *Infant Care in an Urban Community*. London: Allen and Unwin.

Newson, J., and Newson, E. (1976) *Seven Years Old in the Home Environment*. London: Allen and Unwin.

Obeyesekere, G. (1981) *Medusa's Hair: An Essay on Personal Symbols and Religious Experience*. Chicago: Chicago University Press.

O'Brien, M. (1982) Becoming a Lone Father: Differential Patterns and Experiences. In McKee, L. and O'Brien, M. (Eds) *The Father Figure*. London: Tavistock.

Office of Population Censuses and Surveys (1990) *Population Trends*. London: HMSO.

Owen, I.R. (1989) Beyond Carl Rogers: The Work of David Owen. *Holistic Medicine*, **4**, 186–96.

Owens, G., and Jackson, B. (1983) *Adoption and Race: Black, Asian, and Mixed Race Children in White Families*. London: Batsford.

Palazzoli, M.D. *et al.* (1980) *Paradox and Counterparadox*. New York: Jason Aronson.

Parin, P., Morgenthaler, F., and Parin-Mathey, G. (1971) *Fürchte Deinen Nächsten Wie Dich Selbst*. Frankfurt: Suhrkamp.

Parmar, P. (1981) Young Asian Women: A Critique of the Pathological Approach. *Multi-Racial Education*, **9**, No. 3.

*Patterson, C.H. (1978) Cross-Cultural or Intercultural Counselling or Psychotherapy. *International Journal For the Advancement of Counselling*, **1** (3), 231–47.

Pearce, J. (1982) Ethnicity and Family Therapy. In Pearce, J and Friedman, L. (Eds) *Family Therapy: Combining Psychodynamic and Family System Approaches*. New York: Grune and Stratton.

*Pedersen, P.B. (1987) *Handbook of Cross-Cultural Counselling*. New York: Praegar.

*Pedersen, P.B., Draguns, J.G., Lonner, W.J. and Trimble, J.E. (Eds) (1981) *Counselling Across Cultures*, 2nd edn. Honolulu: University of Hawaii Press.

Pedersen, P.B. and Marsella, A. (1980) Ethical Crisis for Cross-Cultural Counselling. *Professional Psychology*, **13**, 492–500.

Perelberg, R.J. (1980) *As Fronterias do Silencio*. Rio de Janeiro: Achiame.

Perelberg, R.J. (1982) Review of Littlewood and Lipsedge's 'Aliens and Alienists'. *Royal Anthropological Institute News*, **50**, 24–5.

Perelberg, R.J. (1983a) Mental Illness, Family and Networks in a London Borough: Two Cases Studies by a Social Anthropologist. *Social Science and Medicine*, **17**, 481–91.

Perelberg, R.J. (1983b) Family and Mental Illness in a London Borough, Unpublished PhD Thesis, University of London.

Perez, M. (1984) Exile: The Chilean Experience. *International Journal of Social Psychiatry*, **30**, 137–61.

Perlman, H.H. (1979) *Relationship: the Art of Helping People*. Chicago: University of Chicago Press.

Phillips, C. (1987) *The European Tribe*. London: Faber and Faber.

Pinderhughes, E.B. (1983) Social Casework. *Journal of Contemporary Social Work*, **4**, 331–7.

Pines, J. (1977) The Study of Racial Images: A Structural Approach. *Screen Education*, **23**, 24–32.

Prince, R. (1964) Indigenous Yoruba Psychiatry. In Kiev (1964a) *op cit*.

Prince, R. (1971) Psychotherapy as a Manipulation of Endogenous Healing Mechanisms. *Transcultural Psychiatric Research Review*, **13**, 115–33.

Pryce, K. (1979) *Endless Pressure: A Study Of West Indian Lifestyles in Bristol*. Harmondsworth: Penguin.

Rachman, S.J. and Wilson, G.T. (1980) *The Effects of Psychological Therapy*, 2nd edn. Oxford: Pergamon Press.

*Rack, P. (1982) *Race, Culture and Mental Disorder*. London: Tavistock.

Rachman, S. (1980) Emotional Processing. *Behaviour Research and Therapy*, **18**.

*Rappoport, R., and Rappoport, R.N. (1982) British Families in Transition. In Rappoport, R.N. *et al.* (Eds), *Families in Britain*. London: Routledge and Kegan Paul.

*Rappoport, R.N. *et al.* (Eds) (1982) *Families in Britain*. London: Routledge and Kegan Paul.

Rasmussen, O.V. (1990) Medical Aspects of Torture. *Danish Medical Bulletin*, **37**, (Supplement 1), 1–88.

Rayner, E. (1971) *Human Development*. London: George Allen and Unwin.

Reynolds, D.K. (1976) *Morita Psychotherapy*. Berkeley: University of California Press.

Rivers, W.H.R. (1924) *Medicine, Magic and Religion*. London: Kegan Paul.

*Robertson, E.E. (1977). *Out of Sight – Not Out of Mind. Studies in Intercultural Social Work*. Birmingham: British Association for Social Work.

*Rogers, C. (1951) Client-centred Therapy. Boston: Houghton-Mifflin.

*Rogers, C. (1961) *On Becoming a Person*. Boston: Houghton-Mifflin.

Rose, D., and Liston, R. (1990) *The Guardian*, 1990.

Rosser, R.M., Birch, S., Bond, H., Denford, J. and Schacter, J. (1987) Five Year Follow Up of Patients Treated With Inpatient Psychotherapy at the Cassell Hospital for Nervous Diseases. *Journal of the Royal Society of Medicine*, **80**.

Rotunno, M. and McGoldrick, M. (1982) Italian Families. In McGoldrick, M. *et al.* (Ed) *Ethnicity and Family Therapy*. New York: Guildford Press.

*Royer, J. (1977) *Black Britains Dilemma: A Medical–Social Transcultural Study of West Indians*. Roseau, Dominica: Tropical Printers.

Russell, D.M. (1988) Language and Psychotherapy. In Comas-Diaz and Griffith *op cit.*

Russell, G. (1983) *The Changing Role of Fathers*. Milton Keynes: Open University Press.

*Salzberger-Wittenberg, I. (1970) *Psycho-Analytic Insight and Relationships – A Kleinian Approach*. London: Routledge and Kegan Paul.

Samouilidis, L. (1978) Psychoanalytic Vicissitudes in Working With Greek Patients. *American Journal of Psychoanalysis*, **38**, 232–3.

Sargant, W. (1957) *Battle for the Mind: A Physiology of Conversion and Brainwashing*. London: Heinemann.

Sartre, J.P. (1948) *Anti-Semite and Jew*. New York: Schocken.

Sartorius, N., Jablensky, A. and Shapiro, R. (1977) Two Year Follow-up of the Patients Included in the WHO International Pilot Study of Schizophrenia. *Psychological Medicine*, **7**, 529–41.

Scheff, T.J. (1979) *Catharsis in Healing, Ritual and Drama*. Berkeley: University of California Press.

Schlapobersky, J. and Bamber, H. (1988) *Torture as the Perversion of a Healing Relationship: Rehabilitation and Therapy with the Victims of Torture and Organised Violence*. Paper presented at the Annual Meeting of the American Association for the Advancement of Science (Boston) pp 1–18. Copies available from the Medical Foundation For the Care of Victims of Torture, 96–98 Grafton Road, London, NW5 3EJ.

Searle, C. (1972) *The Forsaken Lover: White Words and Black People*. London: Routledge and Kegan Paul.

Sedwick, P.Z. (1982) *Psychopolitics*. London: Pluto.

*Shapiro, D.A., Firth-Cozens, J., Stiles, W.B. (1989). The Question of Therapists' Differential Effectiveness – A Sheffield Psychotherapy Project Addendum. *British Journal of Psychiatry*, **154**, 383–5.

Shepherd, M., and Wilkinson, G.L. (1988) Primary Care as the Middle Ground for Psychiatric Epidemiology: Current Status. Editorial. *Psychological Medicine*, **18**, 21.

*Sherwood, R. (n.d.), *The Psychodynamics of Race*. Sussex: The Harvester Press.

Shon, S.P. and Davis, Y. (1982) Asian Families. In McGoldrick, M. *et al.* (Eds) *Ethnicity and Family Therapy*. New York: The Guildford Press.

Shook, E.V. (1985) *Ho'oponopono: Contemporary Uses of a Hawaiian Problem-Solving Process*. Honollulu: East West Center.

Shweder, R.A. (1985) Menstrual Pollution, Soul Loss and The Comparative Study of Emotions. In Kleinman and Good *op cit*.

Simons, R.C. and Hughes, C.C. (Eds) (1985) *The Culture Bound Syndromes: Folk Illnesses of Psychiatric and Anthropological Interest*. Dordrecht: Reidel.

Slobodin, R. (1978) *W.H.R. Rivers*. New York: Columbia University Press.

Sluzki, C. (1979) Migration and Family Conflict. *Family Process*, **18**, 379–90.

Somnier, F.E. and Genefke, I.K. (1986). Psychotherapy for Victims of Torture. *British Journal of Psychiatry*, **149**, pp 323–9.

Spiegel, J.P. (1957) The Resolution of Role Conflict Within the Family. In Greenblatt, M. *et al.* (Eds) *The Patient and the Mental Hospital: Contributions of Research in the Sciences of Social Behaviour*. Glencoe, Illinois: Free Press.

Stanton, M.D. (1981) An Integrated Structural/Strategic Approach to Family Therapy. *Journal of Marital Family Therapy*, **17**. No. 4.

Steinberg, D. (1981) *Using Child Psychiatry*, London: Hodder and Stoughton.

Steinberg, D. (1983) *The Clinical Psychiatry of Adolescence*. Chichester: Wiley.

Steinberg, D. (1986) *The Adolescent Unit: Work and Teamwork in Adolescent Psychiatry*, Chichester: Wiley.

Steinberg, D. (1989) *Interprofessional Consultation: Innovation and Imagination in Working Relationships*. Oxford: Blackwell Scientific Publications.

Steinberg, D. (1991) Achievement in Failure: Working with Staff in Dangerous Situations: A Creative Workshop. International Conference on Children and Death, Athens 1989. In Papadatos, C. and Papadatou, D. (Eds) *Children and Death*, Washington: Hemisphere Publishing.

Steinberg, D. and Hughes, L. (1987) The Emergence of Work-centre Issues in Consultative Work. *Journal of Adolescence*, **10**, 309–16.

Steinberg, D., Wilson, M., and Acharyya, S. (1989) 'My Body Hurts, My Spirit Hurts' – The Relationship between Body, Mind and Soul, A Workshop. *In Proceedings of the Conference on Assessment and Treatment Across Cultures*. London: Nafsiyat, pp. 80–82.

Steinberg, D., and Yule, W. (1985) Consultative Work. In Rutter, M. and Hersov, L. *Child and Adolescent Psychiatry – Modern Approaches*. London: Blackwell Scientific Publications.

Steiner, R. (1975) 'It's a New Kind of Diaspora . . .'. *International Review of Psycho-Analysis*, **16**, 35–78.

Stengel, E. (1939) On Learning a New Language. *International Journal of Psychoanalysis,* **20,** 1–47.

Stigler, J.W., Shweder, R.A., and Herdt, G. (Eds) (1990) *Cultural Psychology.* Cambridge: Cambridge University Press.

*Street, B. (1975) *The Savage in Literature.* London: Routledge and Kegan Paul.

*Sue, D.W. (1981) *Counselling the Culturally Different.* New York: Wiley.

Svendsen, G. (1985). When Dealing With Torture Victims, Social Work Involves the Entire Family. Published in *Socialrudgivern.* English Version available from the International Rehabilitation Centre to Torture Victims, Copenhagen.

Szasz, T. (1971) *The Manufacture of Madness: A Comparative Study of the Inquisition and the Mental Health Movement.* London: Routledge and Kegan Paul.

Taylor, D.C. (1979) The Components of Sickness: Diseases, Illnesses and Predicaments. *Lancet,* **ii,** 1008–10.

Teish, L. (1985) *Jambalaya: The Natural Women's Book of Personal Charms and Practical Rituals.* San Francisco: Harper and Row.

Thomas, A. and Sillen, S. (1972) *Racism and Psychiatry.* New York: Brunner/Mazel.

Timerman, J. (1985) Quoted by Kolff, C.A. and Doan, R.N. Victims of Torture: Two Testimonies. In Stover, E. and Nightingale, E.O. (Eds) *The Breaking of Minds and Bodies* New York: W.H. Freeman, p 53.

Torrey, E.F. (1971) *The Mind Game: Witchdoctors and Psychiatrists.* New York: Emerson Hall.

Townsend, J.M. (1979) Stereotypes of Mental Illness: A Comparison with Ethnic Stereotypes. *Culture, Medicine and Psychiatry,* **3,** 205–29.

Truax, C.B. and Carkhuff, R.R. (1967) *Towards Effective Counselling and Psychotherapy.* Chicago: Chicago Press.

Turner, S.W., and Gorst-Unsworth, C. (1990) Psychological Sequelae of Torture: A Descriptive model. *British Journal of Psychiatry,* **157,** 475–80.

Turner, S.W., and Gorst-Unsworth, C. (1992) Psychological Sequelae of Torture. In Wilson, J., and Raphael, B. (Eds) *The International Handbook of Traumatic Stress Syndromes.* New York: Plenum Press (in press).

Turner, S.W., and Hough, A. (1992) Hyperventilation as a Reaction to Torture. In Wilson, J., and Raphael, B. (Eds) *The International Handbook of Traumatic Stress Syndromes.* New York: Plenum Press (in press).

Turner, V. (1964) An Ndembu Doctor in Practice. In Kiev 1964a *op cit.*

*Twyman, M. (1984) Acting Out. *Journal of the British Association of Psychotherapists.* **20** (15).

Tyler, S.A. (1986) Post-Modern Ethnography. In Clifford, J. and Marcus, G.E. (Eds) *Writing Culture: the Poetics and Politics of Ethnograpy.* Berkeley: University of California Press.

Tyler, P. and Steinberg, D. (1987) *Models for Mental Disorder: Conceptual Models in Psychiatry.* Chichester: Wiley.

Tylor, E.B. (1871) *Primitive Culture.* London: John Murray.

United Nations (1984) *United Nations Convention against Torture and Other Cruel and*

Inhuman or Degrading Treatment or Punishment. New York: Office of Public Information, United Nations.
Utting, W.B. (1990) *Issues of Race and Culture in the Family Placement of Children.* Social Services Inspectorate: Department of Health.

*Vasques-Barquero, J.L., Diez-Manrique, J.F., Pena, C., Quintanal, R.G. *et al.* (1986). Two Stage Design in Community Survey. *British Journal of Psychiatry,* **149,** 88–97.
Velho, G. (1981) *Individualismo e Cultura.* Rio De Janeiro: Zahar.

Wallace, E.R. (1983) *Freud and Anthropology,* New York: International University Press.
Watson, J. (Ed) (1977) *Between Two Cultures: Migrants and Minorities in Britain.* Oxford: Basil Blackwell.
*Westermeyer, J. (1985) Psychiatric Diagnosis Across Cultural Boundaries. *American Journal of Psychiatry,* **142,** 7, 798–805.
*Wilcox, R. (1971) *The Psychological Consequences of Being a Black American.* New York: Wiley.
Wing, J.K., Cooper, J.E., and Sartorius, N. (1974) *Measurement and Classification of Psychiatric Symptoms.* Cambridge: Cambridge University Press.
Winnicott, D. (1975) *Primary Maternal Pre-Occupations. Collected Papers.* London: Tavistock.
Wintrob, R.H., and Harvey, Y.K. (1982) The Self-Awareness Factor in Intercultural Therapy. In Pederson, P.B., Draguns, J.G., Lonner, W.J., and Trimble, J.E. (Eds), *Counselling Across Cultures,* 2nd edn. Honolulu: Hawaii University Press.
Wolin, S.J., and Bennett, L.A. (1984) Family Rituals. *Family Process,* **23,** 401–20.
World Health Organisation (1978) *Mental Disorders: Glossary and Guide to their Classification in Accordance with the Ninth Revision of the International Classification of Disease.* Geneva: World Health Organisation.

*Young, M., and Willmott, P. (1957) *Family and Kinship in East London.* Harmondsworth: Penguin.
Young, M., and Willmott, P.L. (1975) *The Symmetrical Family.* Harmondsworth: Penguin.

*Zwingman, C.A. (1983) *Uprooting and Health: Psychosocial Problems of Students from Abroad.* Geneva: World Health Organisation.

Index